Step by Step

Approach to Fractures

Step by Step

Approach to Fractures

Rahij Anwar
MBBS MS (Orth) [India] MSc (Trauma), MRCS [UK]
Honorary Fellow of Institute of Accident Surgery
Birmingham, UK
Registrar, Trauma and Orthopaedics
Maidstone Hospital, Maidstone (Kent)
United Kingdom

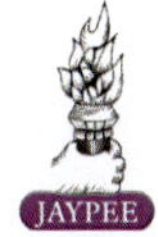

JAYPEE BROTHERS MEDICAL PUBLISHERS
The Health Sciences Publisher
New Delhi | London

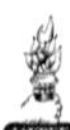

Jaypee Brothers Medical Publishers (P) Ltd

Headquarters
EMCA House
23/23-B, Ansari Road, Daryaganj
New Delhi 110 002, India
Landline: +91-11-23272143, +91-11-23272703
+91-11-23282021, +91-11-23245672
E-mail: jaypee@jaypeebrothers.com

Overseas Office
J.P. Medical Ltd
83 Victoria Street, London
SW1H 0HW (UK)
Phone: +44 20 3170 8910
E-mail: info@jpmedpub.com

Corporate Office
4838/24, Ansari Road, Daryaganj
New Delhi 110 002, India
Phone: +91-11-43574357
Fax: +91-11-43574314
E-mail: jaypee@jaypeebrothers.com

EU GPSR Authorised Representative
Logos Europe, 9 rue Nicolas Poussin
17000, La Rochelle, France
Phone: +33 (0) 6 67 93 73 78
E-mail: contact@logoseurope.eu

Website: www.jaypeebrothers.com
Website: www.jaypeedigital.com

Inquiries for bulk sales may be solicited at: jaypee@jaypeebrothers.com

Step by Step Approach to Fractures

First Edition : 2005

Reprint: 2026
ISBN 978-81-8061-559-7

Printed at: Samrat Offset Pvt. Ltd.

Dedicated to my Uncles

Dr Syed Hasan Iqbal

and

Late Mr Shaheed Uddin Ahmed

PREFACE

The aim of this book is to provide a readily accessible reference for the treatment of fractures. Liberal use of illustrations combined with relevant details in the text will help the reader in remembering and understanding the fracture management clearly. After all, a picture is worth a thousand words!

The book is divided into three sections that systematically cover most of the commonly encountered fractures. In each section, there are chapters covering each region of the body. Important and relevant details about each fracture, are covered. I have tried to include at least one illustration for the common methods of operative management of each fracture.

A word of caution! This book is not aimed to provide a comprehensive review of fractures. All students preparing for orthopaedic postgraduate examinations should refer to the common textbooks for more details.

This book is intended to help all orthopaedic trainees, Accident and Emergency doctors, practicing orthopaedic surgeons, general practitioners, nurses and physiotherapists.

I hope that this book will be of use to the readers, and I appreciate all comments and suggestions.

Rahij Anwar

ACKNOWLEDGEMENTS

'The woods are lovely, dark and deep,
But I have promises to keep,
And miles to go before I sleep,
And miles to go before I sleep.'

—Robert Frost

I am very grateful to the members of the orthopaedic departments at Maidstone and Tunbridge Wells for their enormous support and encouragement during the development of this work. Special thanks are due to Mr KJ Ravikumar for his help and guidance.

I acknowledge the help of Mr SN Anjum for his assistance in the completion of this book.

I am deeply indebted to my friends Dr M Mubashir, Dr S Hasan Harris, Mr Dinesh Govila, Mr M Furqan Shamsi, Dr Shah Alam Khan and all others for their cheerful support.

Thanks to Mr Neil Hallows, deputy editor of the BMA News, for giving me an opportunity to write and for his unfailing encouragement.

I wish to express my gratitude to my orthopaedic teachers (Late Prof AA Khan, Prof SA Sadiq, Prof AA Iraqi, Dr Mohd Zahid, Dr MKA Sherwani and

Dr M Abbas) at the JN Medical College, Aligarh Muslim University, Aligarh (India).

This work would never have been completed without the untiring efforts of my wife, Huma who graciously accepted the long hours needed for writing.

I also wish to acknowledge the help of Miss Sadia Ghani.

I wish to express sincere appreciation to my mother, brothers (Hilal & Talib) and parents-in-law, Mrs and Mr Kabir-ud-Din for their affection and support.

I am also grateful to Shri JP Vij, Chairman and Managing Director and Mr Tarun Duneja, General Manager (Publishing), Jaypee Brothers Medical Publishers (P) Ltd., for their patience and flexibility.

Last but not the least, I am incredibly thankful to my patients who have taught me so much.

CONTENTS

Section 1: Upper Limb

1. **Shoulder and Arm** 3
2. **Elbow and Forearm** 15
3. **Wrist and Hand** 31

Section 2: Lower Limb

4. **Pelvis, Hip and Thigh** 41
5. **Knee and Leg** 59
6. **Ankle and Foot** 67

Section 3: Spine

7. **Spine** 77

Index *85*

Section 1
Upper Limb

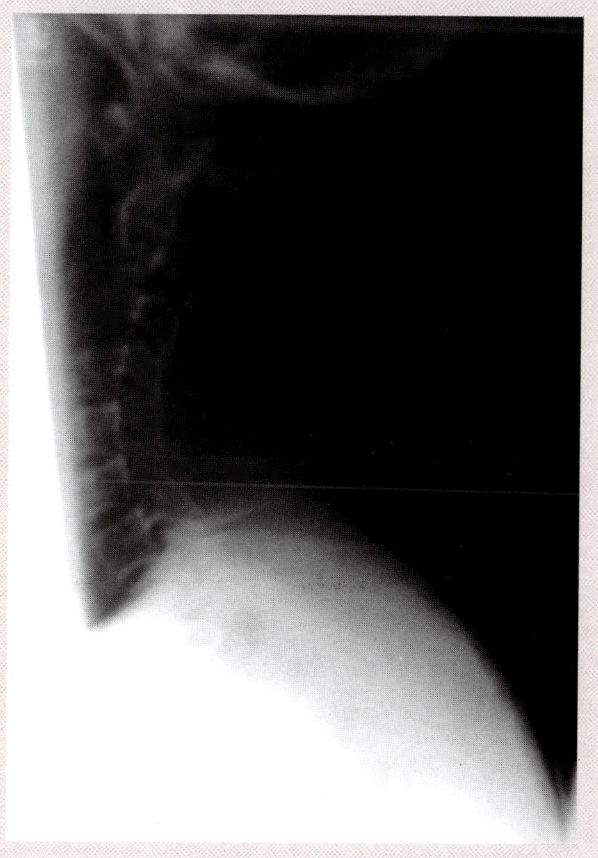

Chapter 1

Shoulder and Arm

FRACTURES OF THE CLAVICLE

Clavicular fractures are caused by a fall on an outstretched hand or from a direct impact at the tip of the shoulder. The medial (proximal) fragment is often pulled upwards due to the action of the sternocleidomastoid muscle and the distal (lateral) fragment displaces inferiorly by the weight of the arm. Associated injuries to the brachial plexus, chest (including rib fractures) and subclavian vesssels may be present. Local tenderness, deformity and painful limitation of movements of the shoulder are important clinical features. A vast majority of these fractures unite following conservative treatment with a sling. Early shoulder mobilisation is encouraged. Open reduction and internal fixation may be considered in certain special situations especially if there is an associated vascular injury or the skin is at risk.

ACROMIOCLAVICULAR JOINT INJURIES

Injuries to the acromioclavicular joint are common after a direct impact at the point of the shoulder. The displacement of the clavicle depends upon the severity of trauma ranging from subluxation to gross disruption of the joint. Associated injuries (e.g. pneumothorax, clavicular fractures, etc.) may be

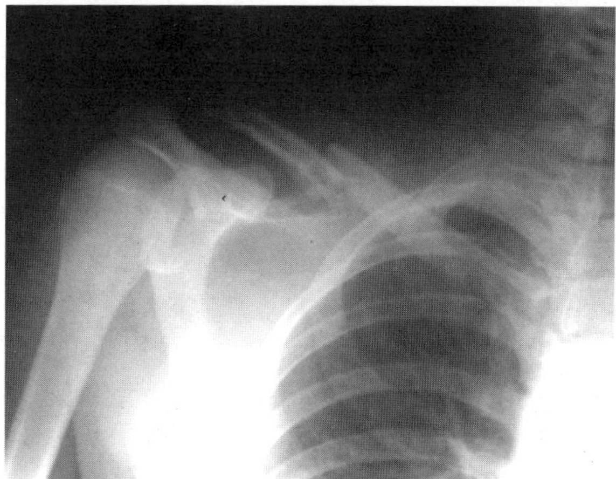

Figure 1.1: AP view of the shoulder showing a fractured clavicle. Most fractures of the clavicular shaft are treated conservatively using a sling

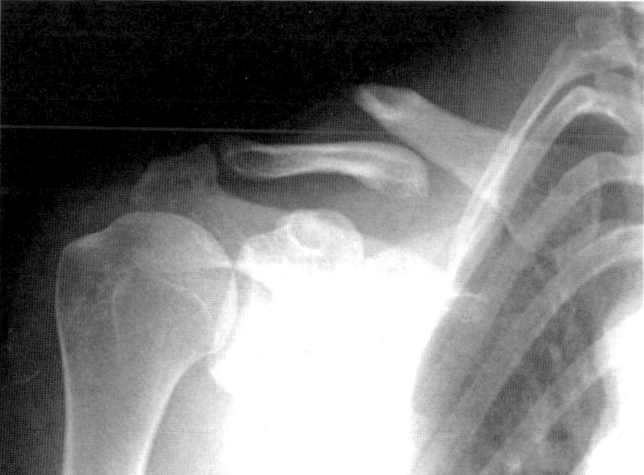

Figure 1.2: AP view of the shoulder showing a non-union of the fractured clavicle. The sharp end of the medial fragment irritated the skin and caused pain

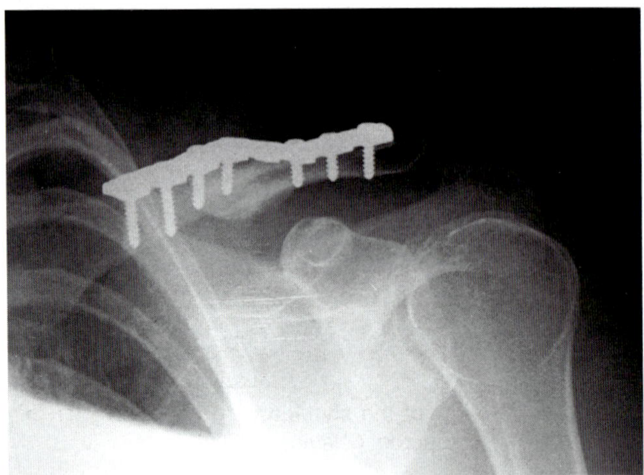

Figure 1.3: AP view of the shoulder. Painful fracture non-union of the clavicle treated with open reduction, internal fixation and bone grafting

present. Minor displacements can be satisfactorily managed conservatively. Open reduction and internal fixation (using a plate, coracoacromial screw or suture) is indicated for the more severe types.

SHOULDER DISLOCATIONS

Dislocations of the shoulder joint usually occur after a fall on an outstretched hand. Most shoulder dislocations are anterior. Other types, posterior and inferior (luxatio erecta), are rare. Deformity of the shoulder is obvious on examination. Axillary nerve (tested by assessing deltoid function and sensations

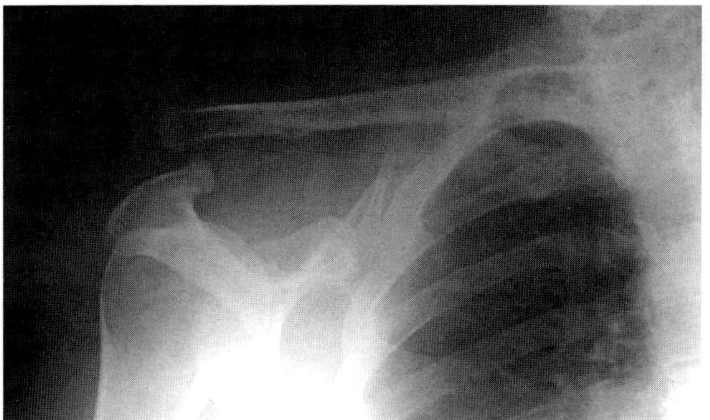

Figure 1.4: AP view of the shoulder showing disruption of the acromioclavicular joint

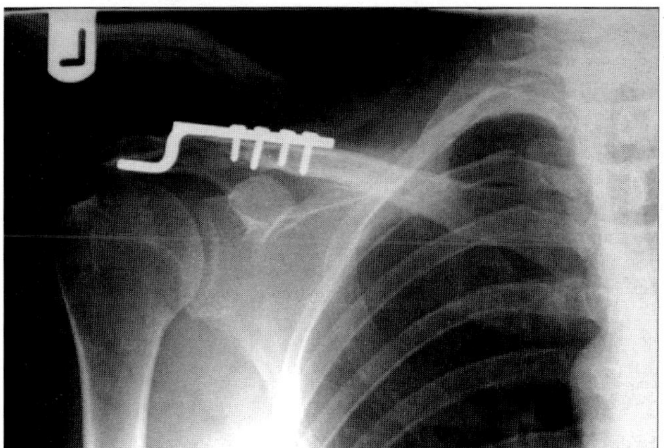

Figure 1.5: AP view of the shoulder showing a disrupted acromioclavicular joint stabilised by open reduction and internal fixation using a hook plate

in the 'regimental badge' area) may be involved. Associated injuries like fractures of the proximal humerus (e.g. greater tuberosity) may be present. Reduction is achieved by manipulation under intravenous sedation or general anaesthetic. Surgery is reserved for recurrent dislocations or in cases associated with significantly displaced fractures, especially in young patients.

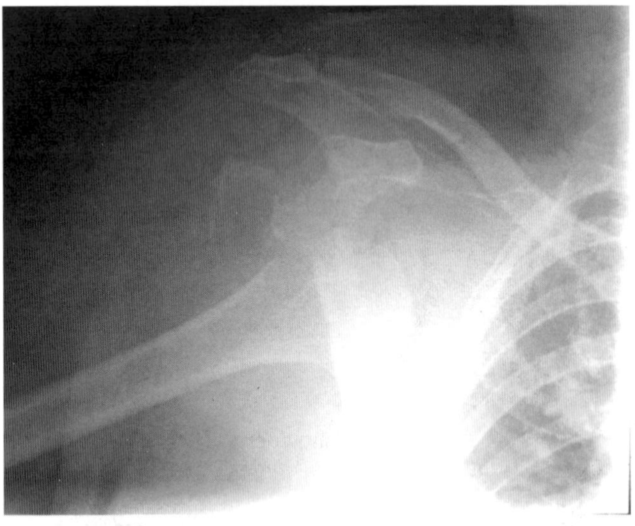

Figure 1.6: AP view of the shoulder showing anterior dislocation of the humeral head associated with a fracture of the greater tuberosity

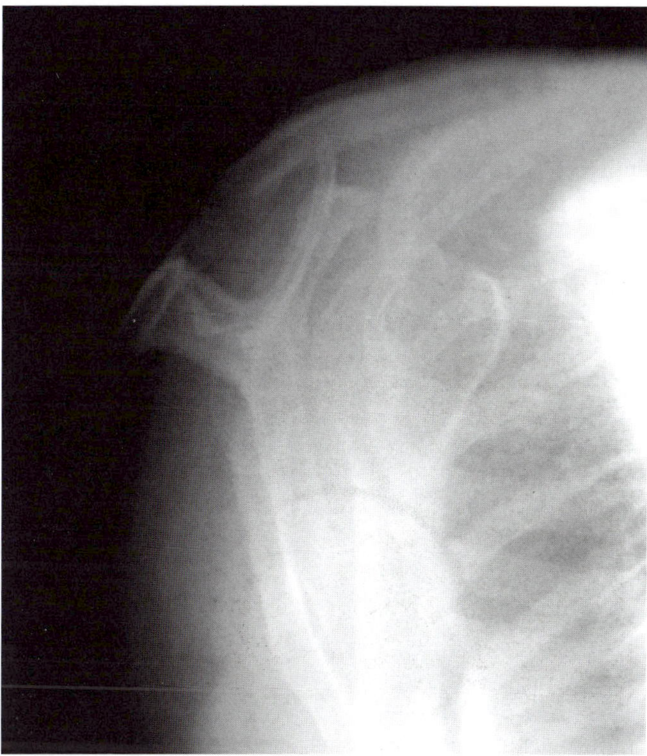

Figure 1.7: Y view of the shoulder showing an anterior dislocation of the humeral head

PROXIMAL HUMERAL FRACTURES

Fractures of the proximal humerus commonly occur in elderly patients, following trivial falls. They may be associated with subluxation or dislocation of the shoulder joint, axillary nerve involvement, chest injuries, etc. Undisplaced or minimally displaced fractures can be satisfactorily treated with a collar and cuff sling. Operative treatment (ORIF/Hemiarthroplasty) is reserved for grossly displaced fractures or those with joint involvement.

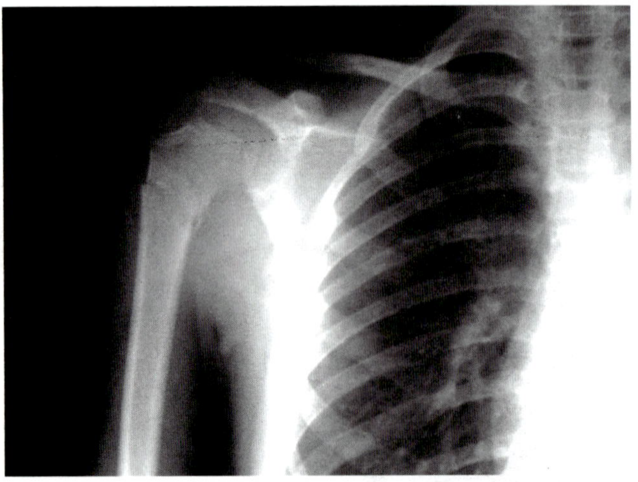

Figure 1.8: Undisplaced or minimally displaced fractures of the proximal humerus can be satisfactorily treated conservatively

FRACTURES OF THE HUMERAL SHAFT

Fractures of the humeral shaft occur following violent trauma (e.g. road traffic accidents). The radial nerve is involved in about 10% cases. Conservative treatment (functional brace or plaster slab) is indicated for a

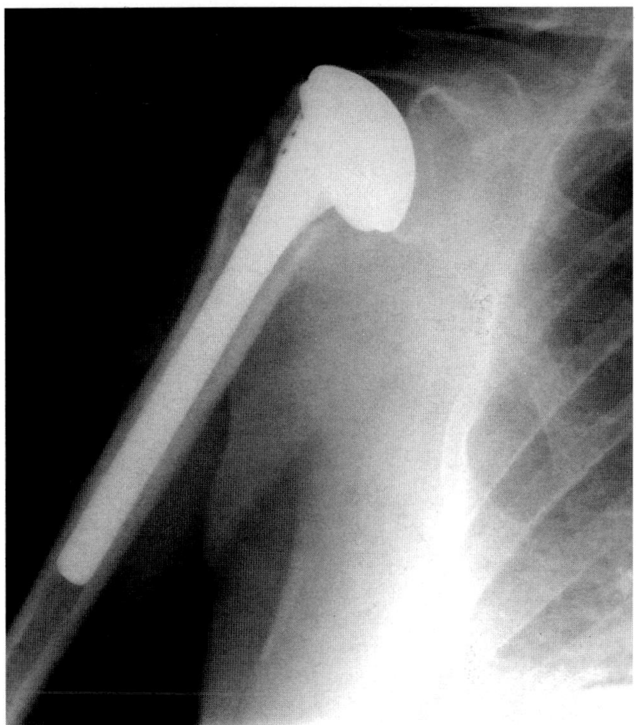

Figure 1.9: AP view showing a hemiarthroplasty (Neer's prosthesis) of the right shoulder following a comminuted fracture of the proximal humerus

majority of the fractures. Internal fixation (Intramedullary nailing or plating) is advisable if conservative treatment fails. Non-union is an important complication.

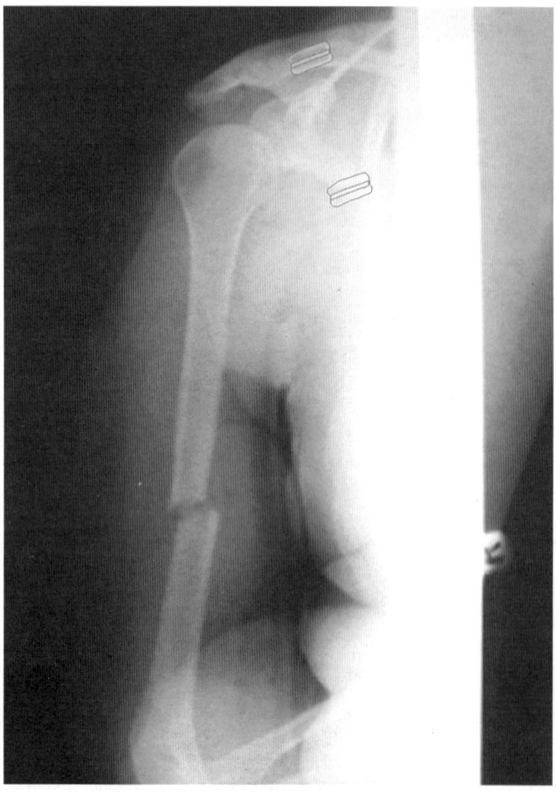

Figure 1.10: A trial of conservative treatment should be given for all humeral shaft fractures with acceptable alignment

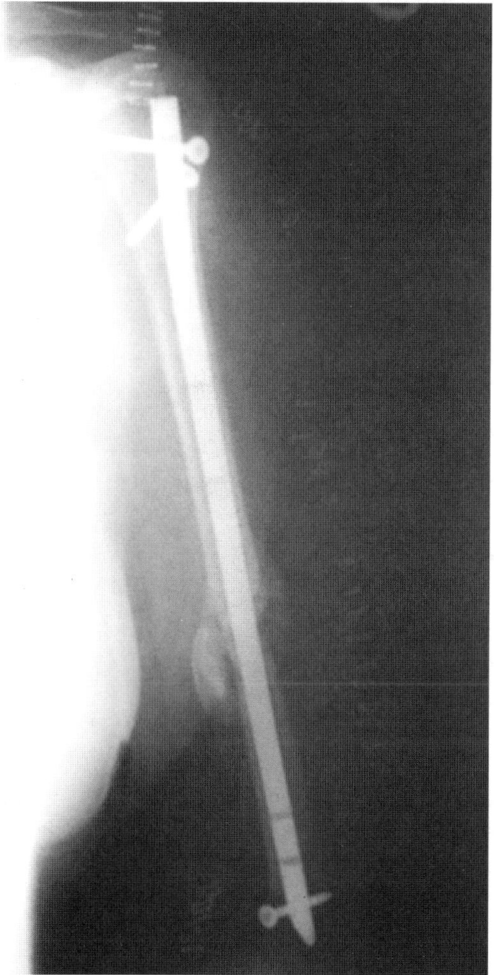

Figure 1.11: AP view of the arm showing an united fracture of the shaft of the humerus treated with intramedullary nailing and bone grafting

CHAPTER 2

Elbow and Forearm

SUPRACONDYLAR FRACTURES OF THE HUMERUS

Supracondylar fractures are common in children. They occur following a fall on an outstretched hand. Gross displacement causes pain, swelling and deformity of the elbow. Examination should include a careful assessment of the function of the peripheral nerves and vessels. Displaced fractures almost always require manipulation plus/minus stabilisation with K-wires. Compartment syndrome, nerve palsies and malunion are important complications.

FRACTURES OF THE LATERAL CONDYLE

Fractures of the lateral condyle occur as a result of indirect trauma to the extended elbow. All displaced fractures should be manipulated and internally fixed using K-wires. The growing child develops progressive valgus deformity and ulnar nerve palsy if the fracture is not reduced or stabilised properly.

INTERCONDYLAR FRACTURES

Impaction of ulna over the trochlea following indirect trauma splits the condyles and disrupts the articulates surface. Anatomical reduction and internal fixation

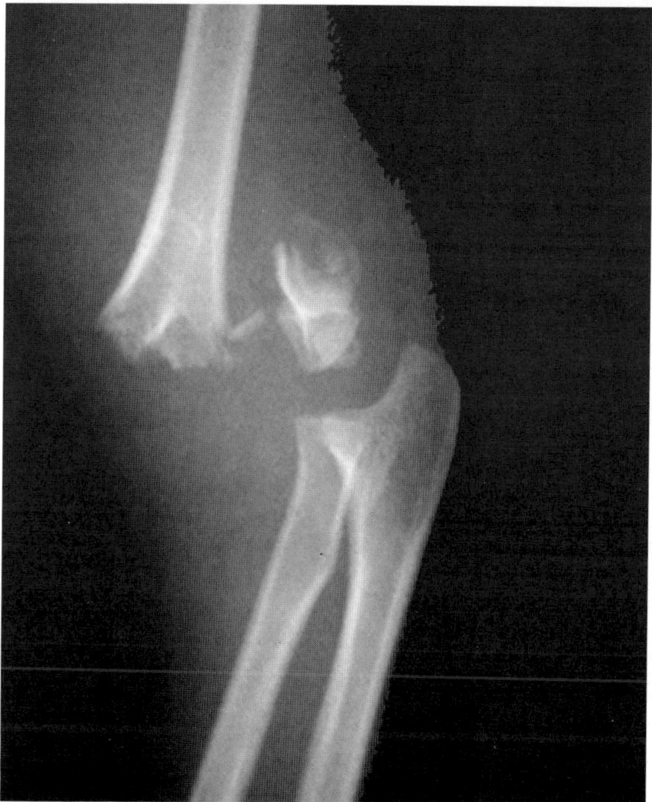

Figure 2.1: Displaced supracondylar fractures of the humerus are common in children

(plates and screws) is often indicated. This is carried-out through a transolecranon or triceps splitting approach. Joint stiffness is common.

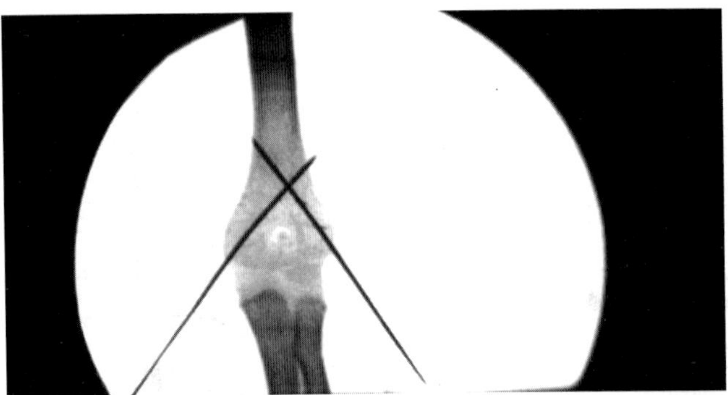

Figure 2.2: AP view of the elbow showing a displaced supracondylar fracture stabilised with two cross K-wires after manipulation

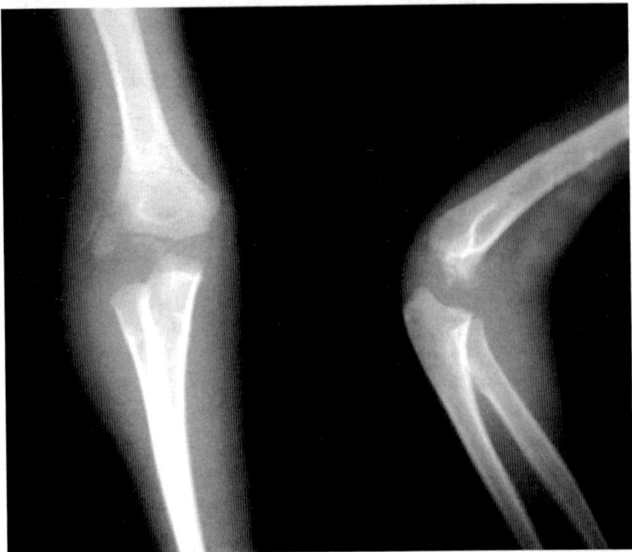

Figure 2.3: AP and lateral views of the elbow showing a displaced fracture of the lateral condyle

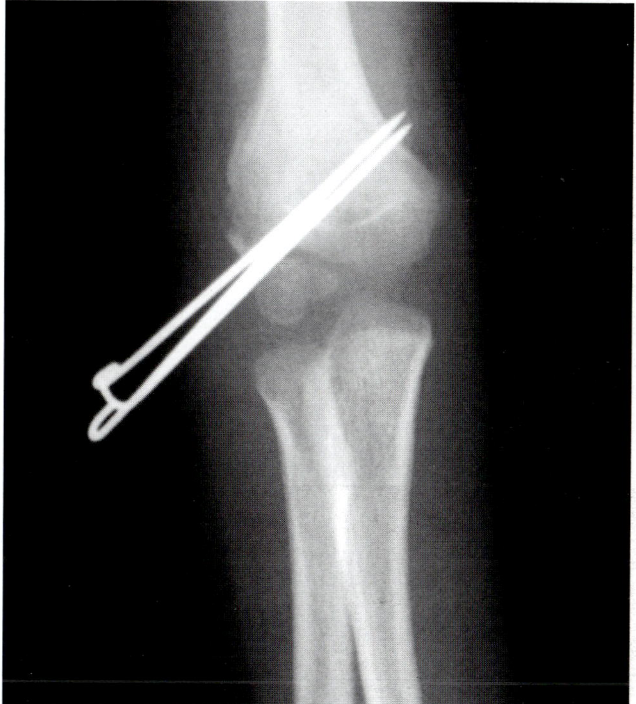

Figure 2.4: Fracture of the lateral condyle stabilised with K-wires

ELBOW DISLOCATIONS

Elbow dislocations result from a fall on an extended elbow. In children, medial epicondyle may avulse and come to lie in the joint. Immediate reduction should be performed. Early motion is advisable.

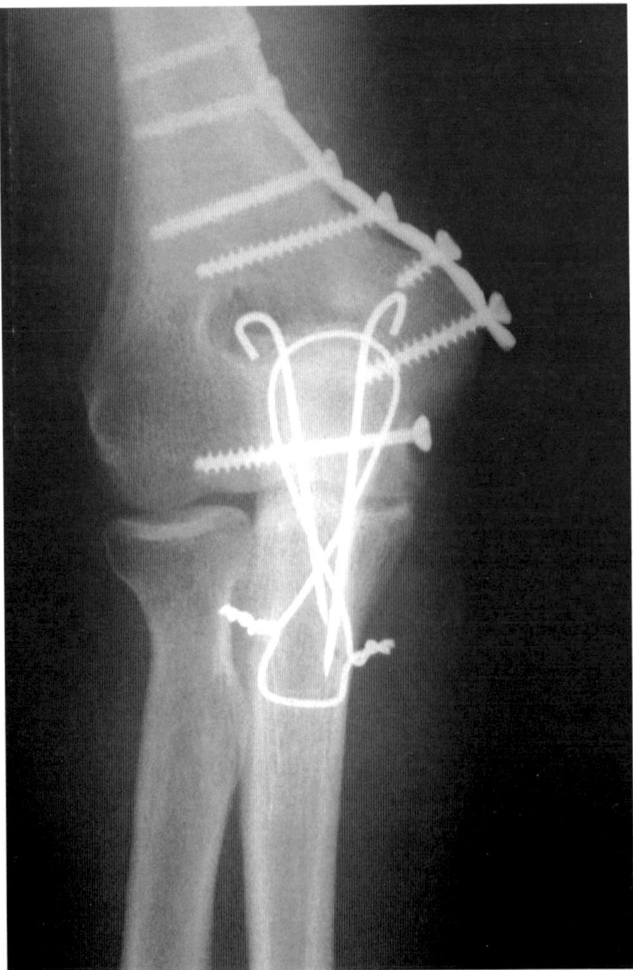

Figure 2.5: AP view of the elbow showing an intercondylar fracture of the humerus treated with internal fixation through the transolecranon approach

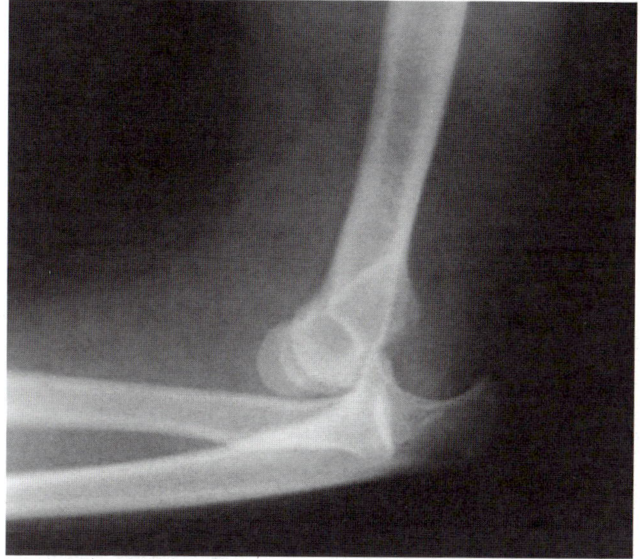

Figure 2.6: Lateral view of a dislocated elbow

OLECRANON FRACTURES

A fall on the outstretched hand combined with the pull of the triceps causes an oblique or transverse fracture of the olecranon. Most fractures are treated with anatomical reduction and internal fixation (Tension band wiring or plating). Early motion is encouraged.

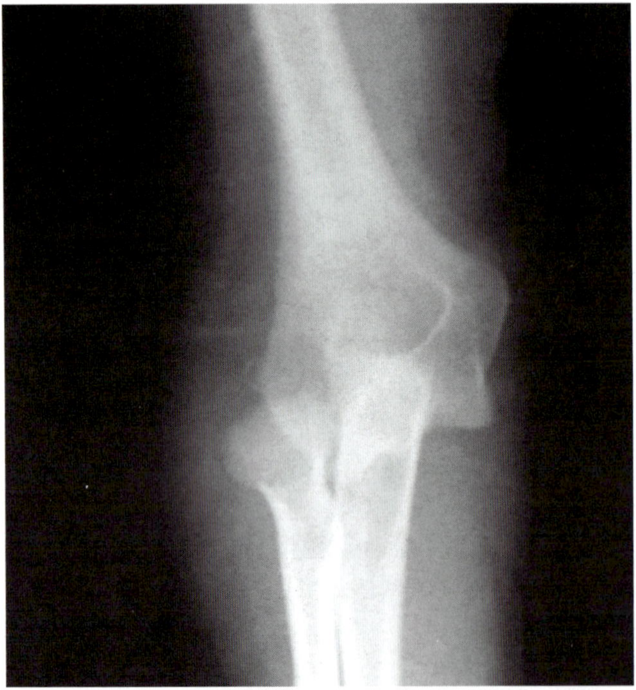

Figure 2.7: AP view of a dislocated elbow

RADIAL HEAD FRACTURES

Fractures of the radial head occur following a fall on the outstretched hand. Other associated injuries like elbow dislocations, olecranon fractures, etc. may also be present. Local tenderness and limitation of movements are common findings on examination. Assessment of elbow stability is important. Most

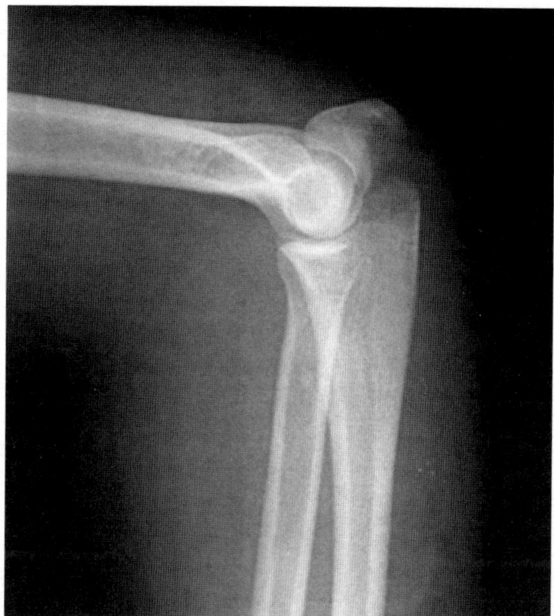

Figure 2.8: Lateral view of the elbow showing a displaced fracture of the olecranon

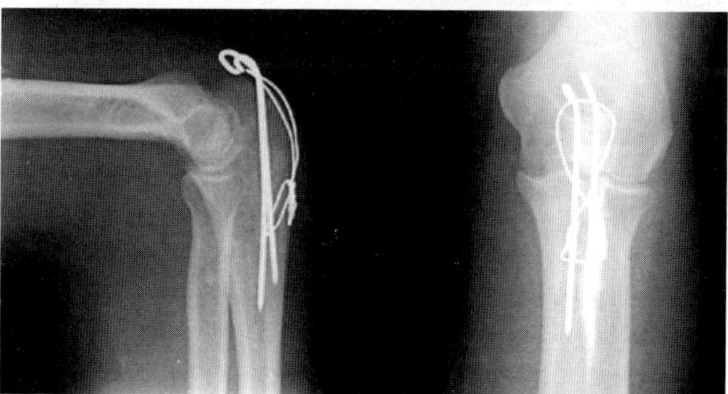

Figure 2.9: AP and lateral views of the elbow showing union of the fractured olecranon following treatment with 'Tension band wiring'

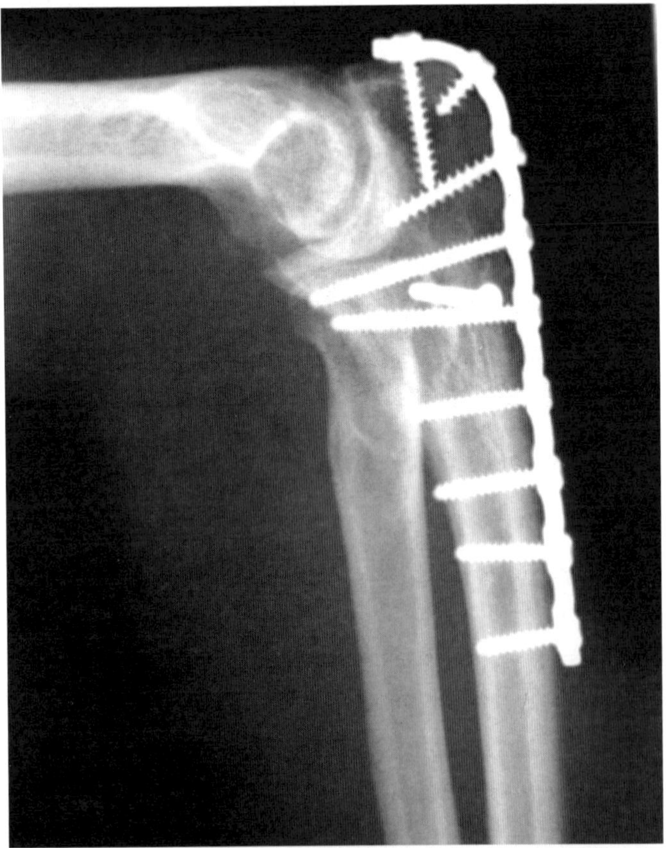

Figure 2.10: Lateral view of the elbow showing fixation of olecranon with a reconstruction plate. The original fracture of the olecranon was too comminuted to be treated with 'Tension band wiring'

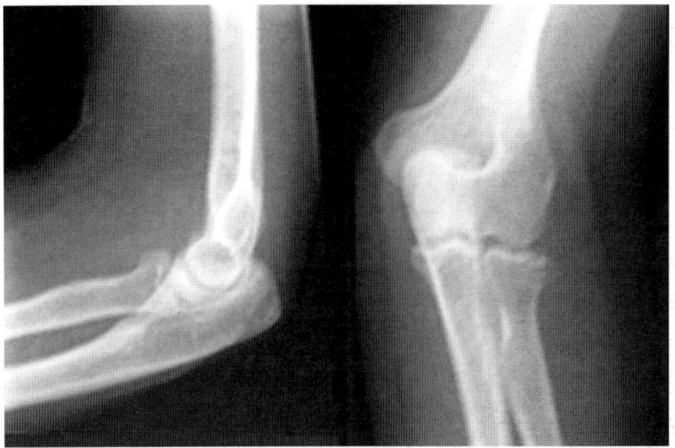

Figure 2.11: AP and lateral views of the elbow showing a minimally displaced fracture of the radial head

fractures are treated conservatively with a sling and early excercises. Open reduction and internal fixation is indicated for displaced fractures in young patients. Excision/prosthetic replacement of the capital fragment is advised for severely comminuted fractures. Early motion should be encouraged to avoid elbow stiffness.

Monteggia's Fracture

A fracture of the proximal ulna associated with a dislocation of the radial head (disruption of the superior radioulnar joint).

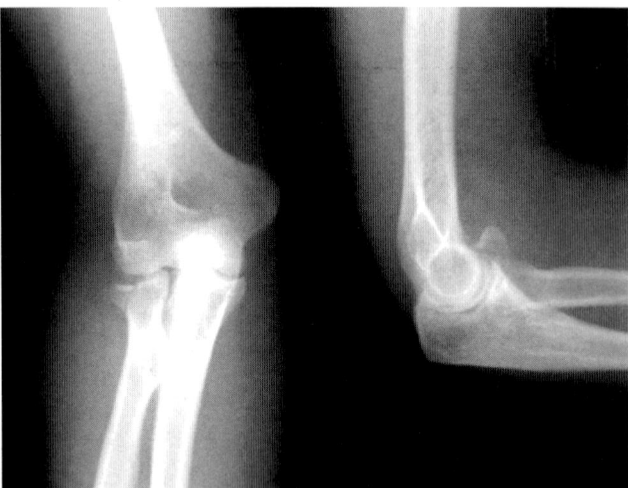

Figure 2.12: AP and lateral views of the elbow showing a significantly displaced fracture of the radial head

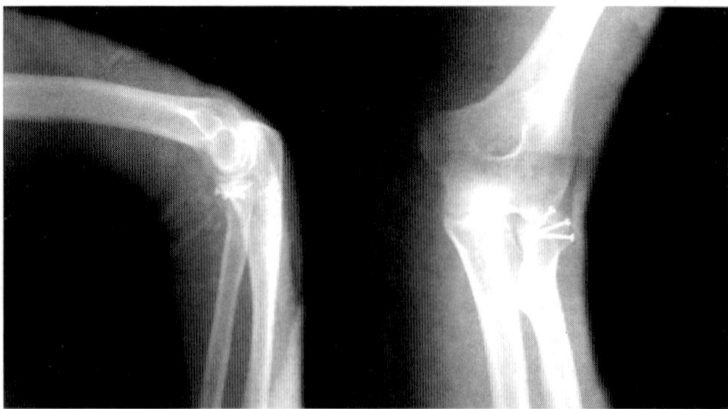

Figure 2.13: AP and lateral views of the elbow showing fixations of a radial head fracture with multiple screws

Galeazzi's Fracture

A fracture of the shaft of the radius associated with a dislocation of the inferior radioulnar joint.

Essex-Lopresti Lesion

A fracture of the radial head associated with a disruption of the interosseous membrane and inferior radioulnar joint.

Nightstick Fracture

A fracture of the distal ulna as a result of direct trauma.

Greenstick Fracture

A diaphyseal fracture associated with a unicortical disruption or 'buckling' of the cortex. Common in children and union is almost certain.

DIAPHYSEAL FRACTURES OF THE RADIUS AND ULNA

Diaphyseal fractures of the forearm bones may occur as a result of both direct and indirect mechanisms. Careful assessment of the wrist and elbow is essential to rule out the involvement of the superior and inferior radioulnar joints. Undisplaced fractures can be

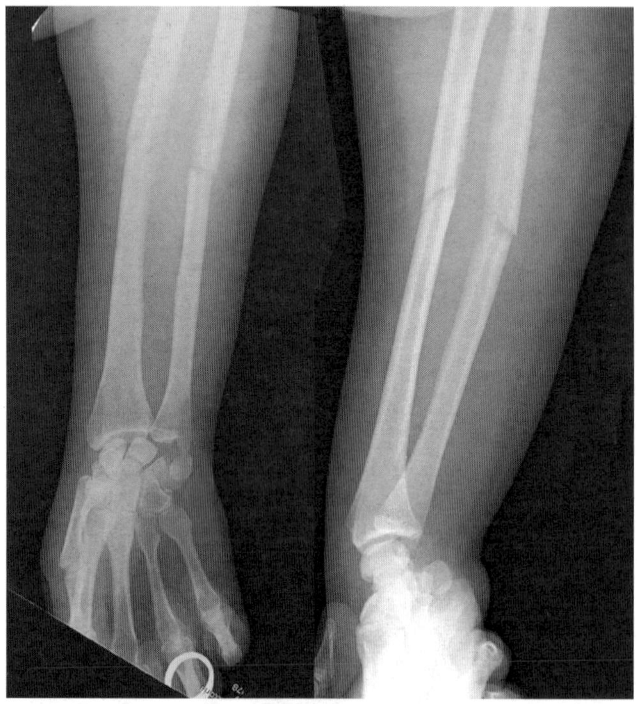

Figure 2.14: AP and lateral views of the forearm showing fracture of the shaft of the radius and ulna

satisfactorily treated with an above elbow cast. Most displaced fractures require open reduction and internal fixation (plating). Some surgeons prefer to use flexible intramedullary nails (Nancy nails) in children.

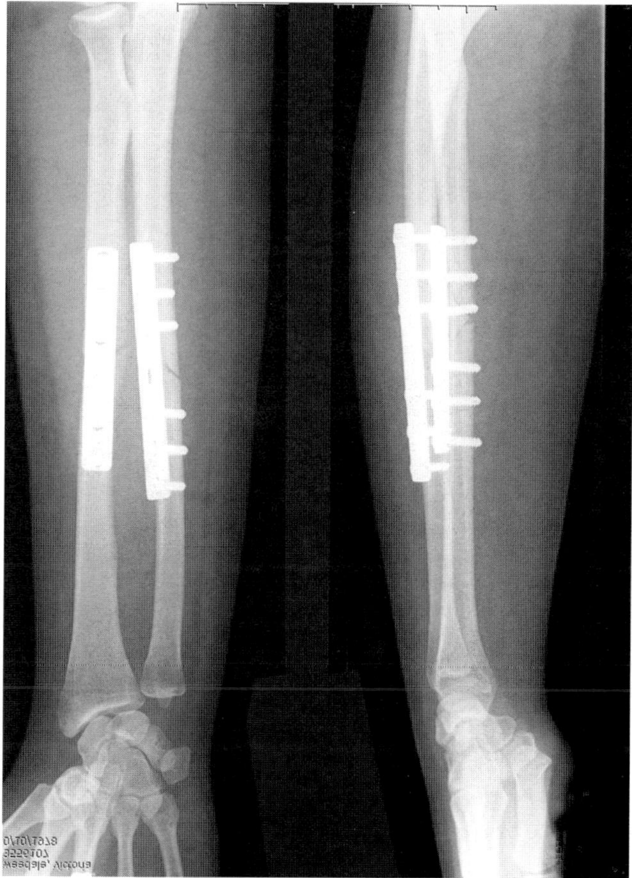

Figure 2.15: Displaced fractures of the radius and ulna often require open reduction and internal fixation

CHAPTER 3

Wrist and Hand

DISTAL RADIUS FRACTURES

Fractures of the distal radius usually occur in the elderly age group due to osteoporosis. A fall on an outstretched hand is the common mechanism of injury. The type of deformity (e.g. dinner fork) depends upon the direction of displacement. Most undisplaced fractures are satisfactorily treated with plaster cast immobilisation. However, manipulation plus/minus K-wiring is often necessary for significantly displaced fractures. Smith's (reversed Colles') and Barton's fractures frequently require open reduction and internal fixation (Buttress plating).

Eponyms

Colles' Fracture

An extra-articular fracture of the distal radius associated with impaction and dorsolateral displacement resulting in the typical 'dinner fork' deformity of the wrist.

Smith's Fracture

An extra-articular fracture of the distal radius associated with volar displacement (reversed Colles'). This type of fracture is caused by a fall with wrist in palmar flexion. Open reduction and internal fixation is often necessary.

Barton's Fracture

An intra-articular fracture of the distal radius associated with volar or dorsal subluxation of the wrist. Operative treatment is necessary for restoration of the anatomy.

Chauffeur's Fracture

A fracture of the radial styloid process.

Scaphoid Fractures

Scaphoid fractures commonly occur following a fall on the outstretched hand. Tenderness in the anatomical snuff box is an important feature. Associated perilunate disruptions injuries are common, especially with high velocity trauma. Immobilisation is recommended for cases with a clinical suspicion even if the radiological examination does not show a clear fracture. Identification of the fracture is easier if the X-rays are repeated couple of weeks after the injury.

Undisplaced fractures should be immobilised in a 'scaphoid cast' for at least six weeks. Displaced fractures or those with a significant gap at the fracture site are often treated with percutaneous screws

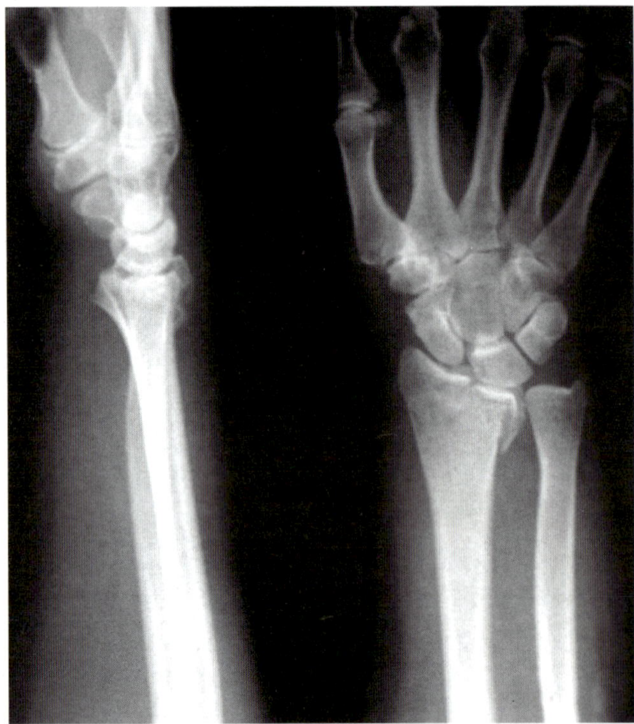

Figure 3.1: AP and lateral views of the wrist showing a fracture of the distal radius with intra-articular extension. Note the step in the articular surface

(Herbert or Acutrek). Sometimes scaphoid fractures fail to unite even with internal fixation.

FRACTURES OF THE METACARPAL

The metacarpal may fracture at any level. Injuries to fifth metacarpal are common. Fracture of the neck of

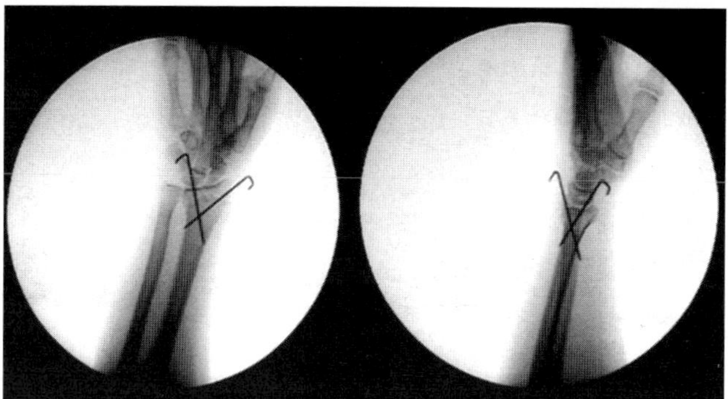

Figure 3.2: AP and lateral views of the wrist showing fixation of a distal radius fractures with K-wires

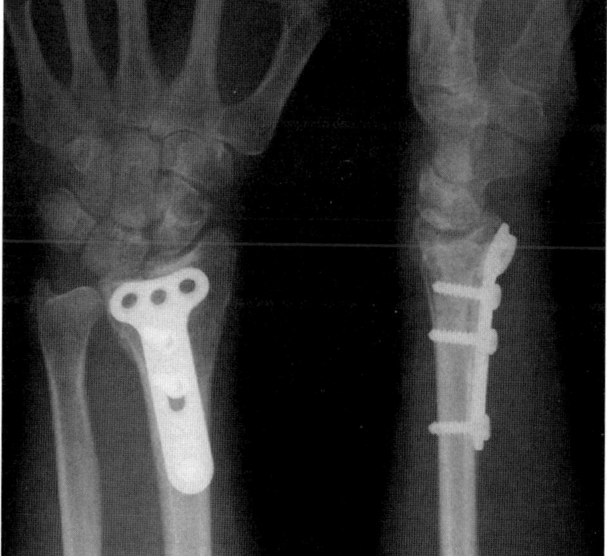

Figure 3.3: AP and lateral views of the wrist. Distal radius fractures, especially those with volar displacement and/or intra-articular involvement (e.g. Smith's or Barton's fracture) often require buttress plating to maintain the position of the fragments

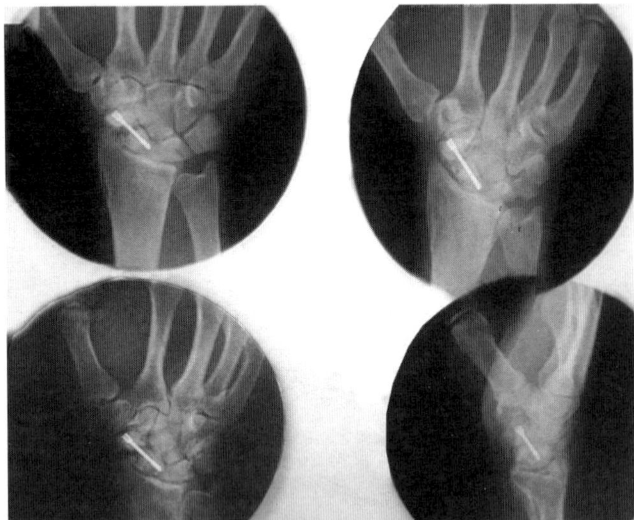

Figure 3.4: Scaphoid views of the wrist showing a non-union of the fractured scaphoid which was initially fixed with a percutaneous screw

the fifth metacarpal (Boxer's fracture) occurs when the hand hits something while closed into a fist.

Examination of the affected ray for rotational and angular deformity is important. The distal fragment is often angulated volarly. Manipulation and internal fixation with K-wires is necessary if the deformity is significant. However, most metacarpal fractures are conservatively treated ('neighbour strapping' of the fingers). Early motion prevents stiffness.

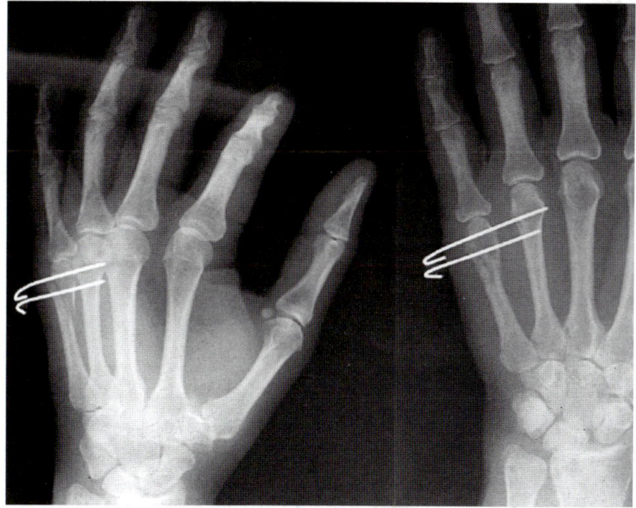

Figure 3.5: AP and oblique views of the hand showing fixation of an oblique (unstable) fracture of the fifth metacarpal stabilised with two transverse K-wires

PHALANGEAL FRACTURES

Injuries to the phalanges occur following a direct impact or a twisting injury.

Most phalangeal fractures can be satisfactorily treated with 'neighbour strapping' (immobilising the injured finger and its neighbour together). However, operative intervention (usually manipulation and K-wiring/screws) is necessary if the fracture configuration is unstable or if there is intra-articular involvement. Stiffness is avoided by early motion.

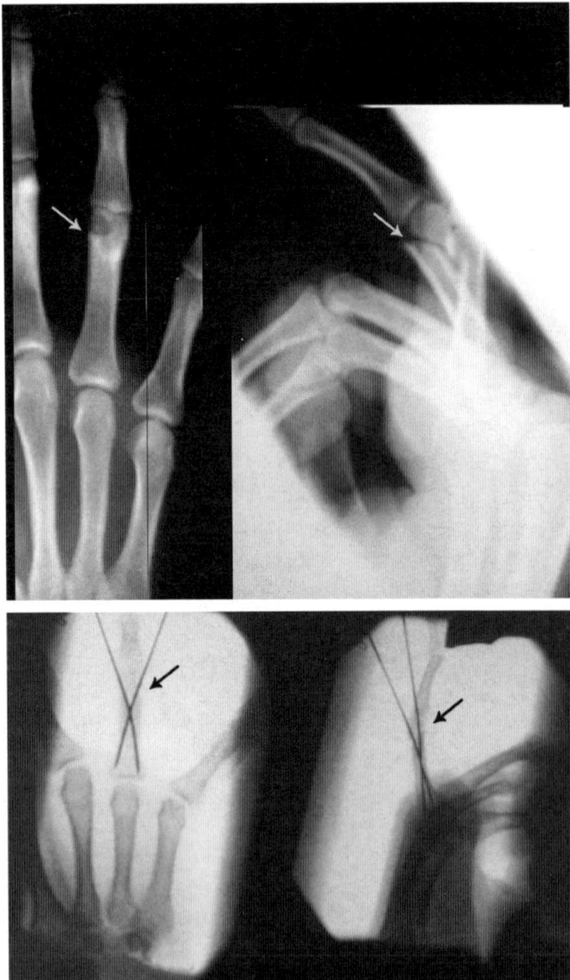

Figure 3.6: AP and lateral views of the ring finger showing a highly unstable oblique fracture of the neck of proximal phalanx (arrow) fixed with two cross K-wires

Section 2
Lower Limb

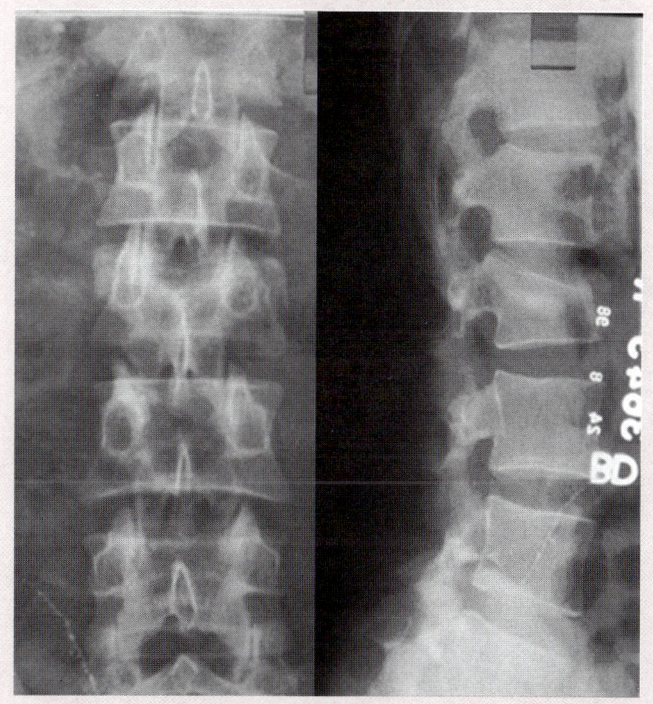

CHAPTER 4

Pelvis, Hip and Thigh

PELVIC FRACTURES

All major pelvic disruptions are associated with high velocity trauma (road traffic accidents, heavy falls, etc.). Simple pubic rami fractures occur with a high frequency in the elderly age group after trivial falls and are usually related to osteoporosis.

Major pelvic disruptions are often associated with hypovolaemia due to the involvement of the pelvic vessels. Injuries to the pelvic viscera, head, chest,

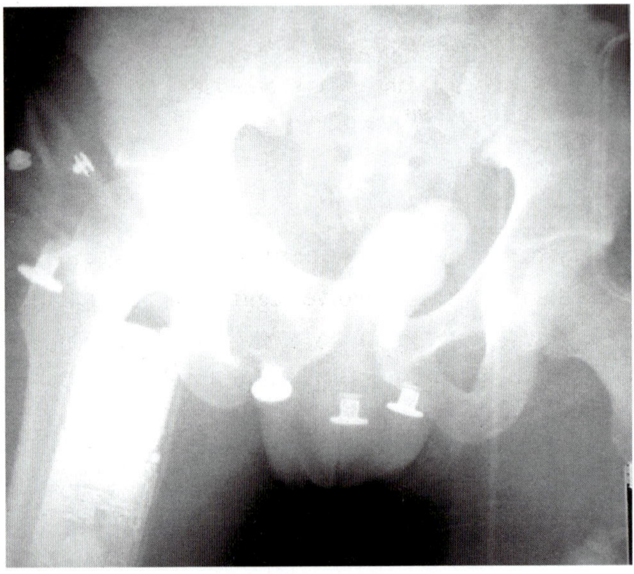

Figure 4.1: An 'Open Book' pelvic injury showing separation of symphysis pubis

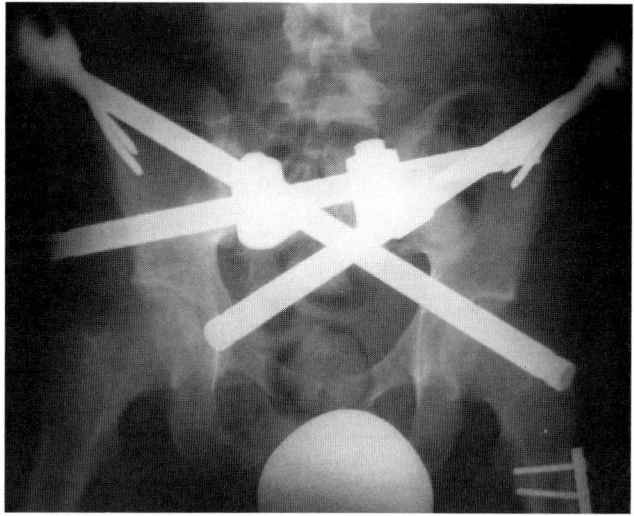

Figure 4.2: AP view of the pelvis showing reduction and fixation of a pelvic injury with an external fixator – a life saving procedure

abdomen and other body parts may also been seen. Immediate treatment involves aggressive resuscitation. Urgent application of an external fixator aids in controlling the haemorrhage and stabilization of the fractures. Internal fixation is often necessary in displaced fractures involving the acetabulum, sacroiliac joint and symphysis pubis. Most undisplaced or minimally displaced fractures are treated conservatively in the absence of pelvic complications.

FRACTURES OF THE HIP

Femoral Neck Fractures

Fractures of the femoral neck are frequently seen in the elderly age group due to osteoporosis. They usually result from trivial falls. Shortening and external rotation of the affected leg are common findings on examination.

Femoral neck fractures may be intracapsular or extracapsular. Hemiarthroplasty (Austin Moore's/ Thompson's/Bipolar prosthesis) is indicated for a vast majority of the displaced intracapsular fractures. Undisplaced or minimally displaced intracapsular fractures are fixed with cannulated screws. Undisplaced unicortical fractures can also be treated conservatively.

Dynamic hip screw fixation (DHS) is the treatment of choice for all extracapsular fractures. However, some intramedullary devices (e.g. proximal femoral nail) may be used if the fracture configuration is unstable.

Non-union, Malunion, avascular necrosis, varus collapse and secondary osteoarthritis are important complications.

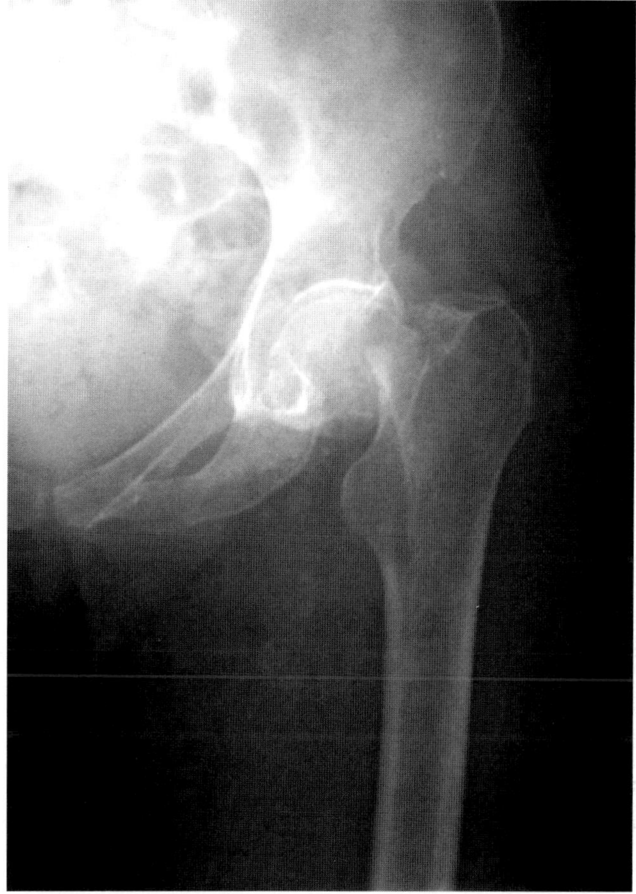

Figure 4.3: AP view of the hip showing a displaced intracapsular fracture of the femoral neck

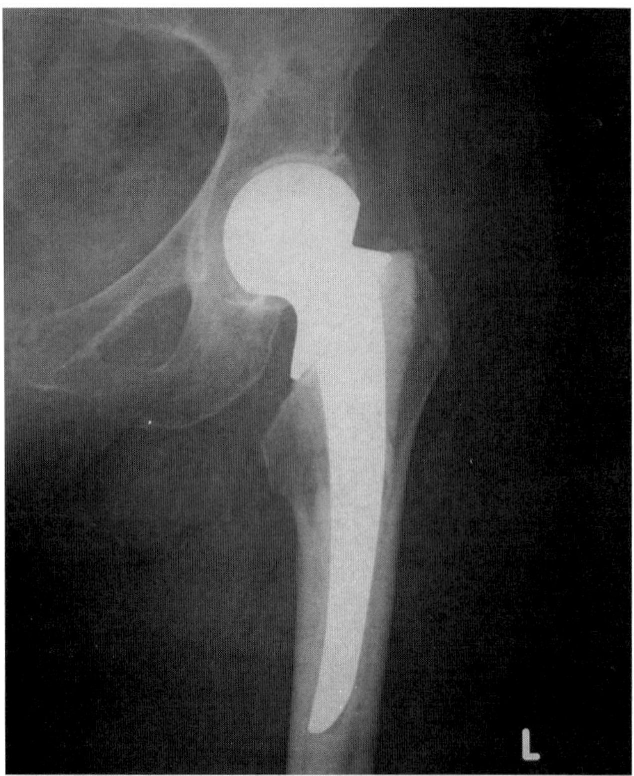

Figure 4.4: AP view of the hip showing a hemiarthroplasty using a cemented Thompson's prosthesis following an intracapsular fracture of the femoral neck

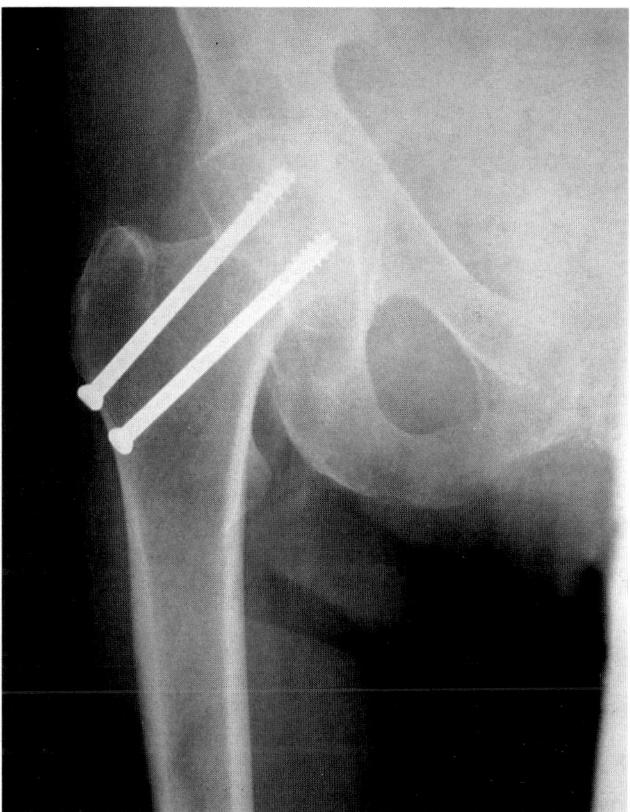

Figure 4.5: AP view of the hip showing an undisplaced intracapsular femoral neck fracture fixed with two cannulated screws

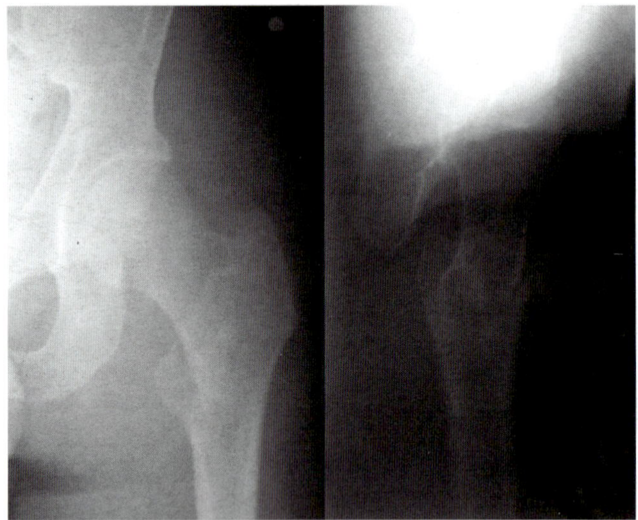

Figure 4.6: AP and lateral views of the hip showing a minimally displaced intertrochanteric fracture

HIP DISLOCATIONS

About 80% of hip dislocations are posterior. The anterior and central types are relatively uncommon. Dislocations occur in response to a violent force (e.g. dashboard injury in a road traffic accident). The limb is shortened, adducted, flexed and internally rotated in a posterior dislocation. However, the deformity is reversed in the anterior type (shortening, flexion, abduction and external rotation). Sciatic nerve involvement may be present in about 10% of cases.

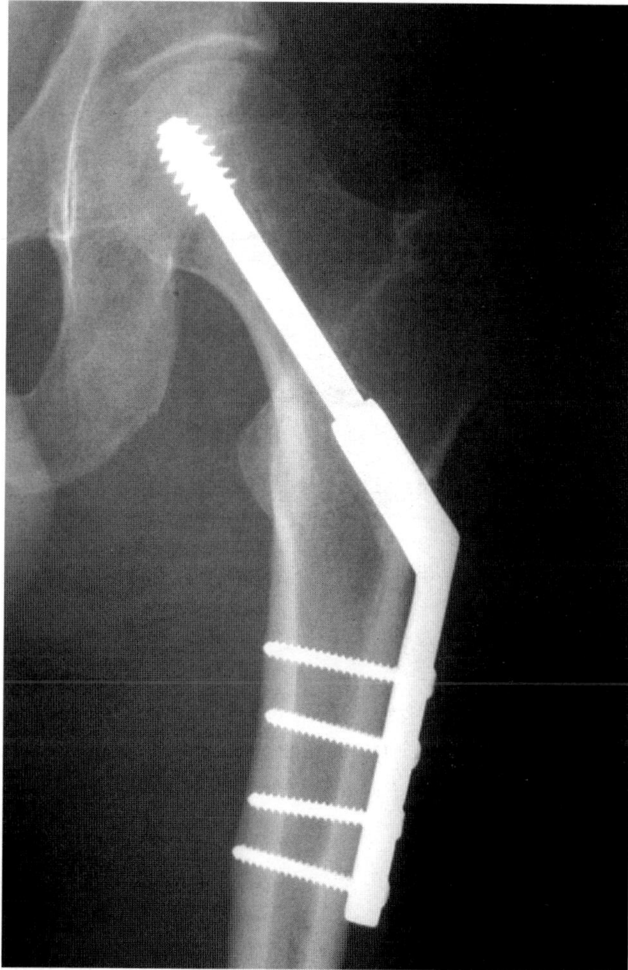

Figure 4.7: AP view of the hip showing union of an extracapsular (intertrochanteric) fracture of the femoral neck following treatment with a dynamic hip screw

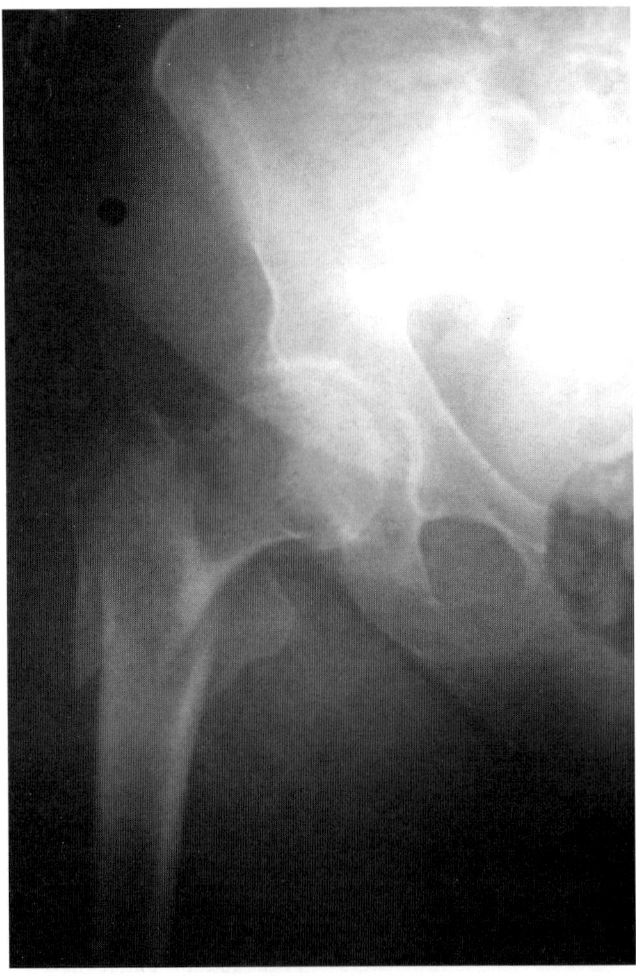

Figure 4.8: AP view of the hip showing an unstable Intertrochanteric fracture

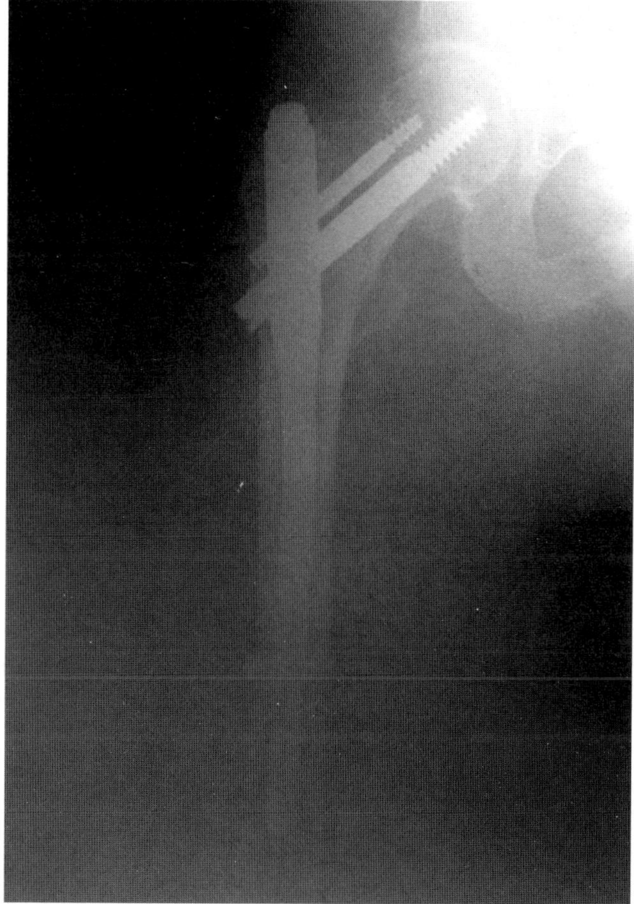

Figure 4.9: AP view of the hip showing fixation of an unstable proximal femoral fracture with a reconstruction nail

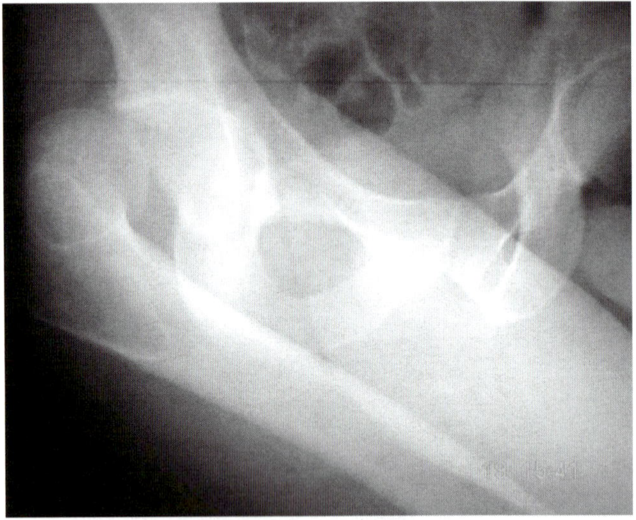

Figure 4.10: AP view of the pelvis showing a posterior dislocation of the right hip. The leg is flexed, adducted and internally rotated

Closed manipulation under intravenous sedation or general anaesthetic is often successful. Very rarely, open reduction may be required. Early mobilisation should be encouraged. Sciatic nerve injury, avascular necrosis and osteoarthritis are important complications.

FRACTURES OF THE FEMORAL SHAFT

Most fractures of the femoral shaft occur as a result of violent trauma (e.g. road traffic accidents). They

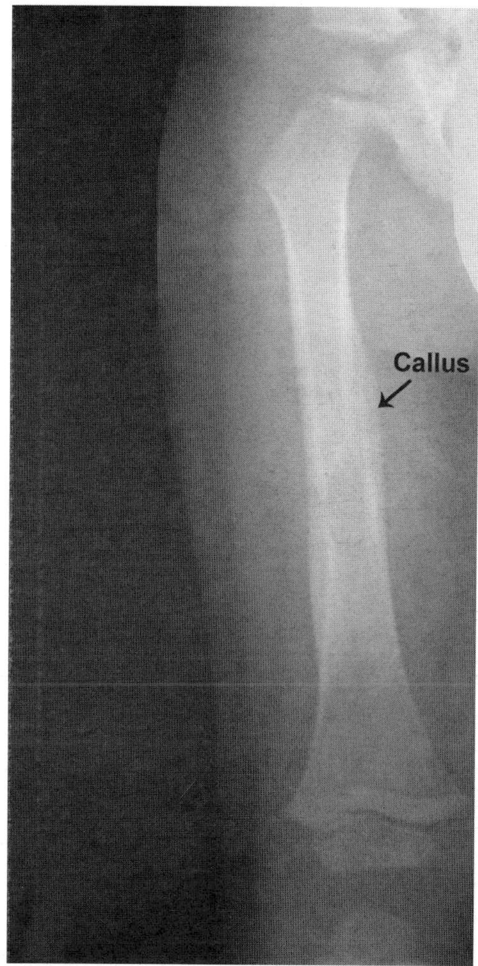

Figure 4.11: Fractures of the femoral shaft in children unite satisfactorily if the alignment is maintained with a plaster spica or traction

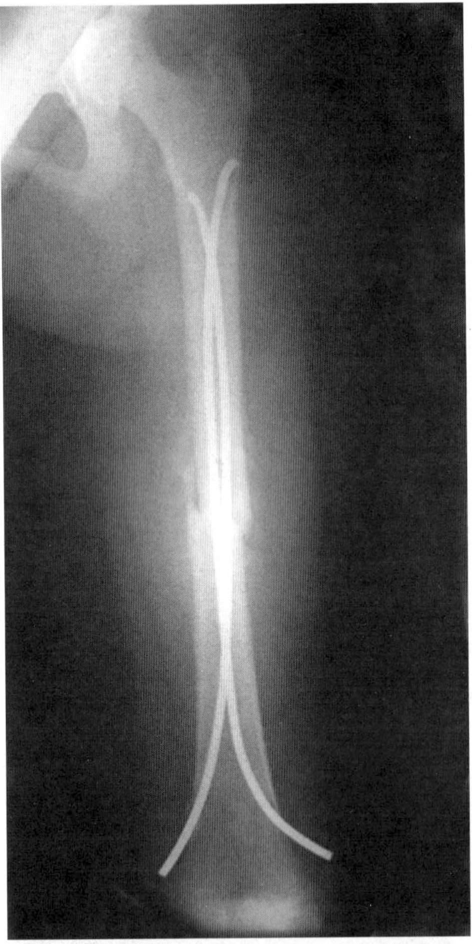

Figure 4.12: Markedly displaced and unstable femoral shaft fractures can be stabilised with flexible intramedullary nails (Nancy)

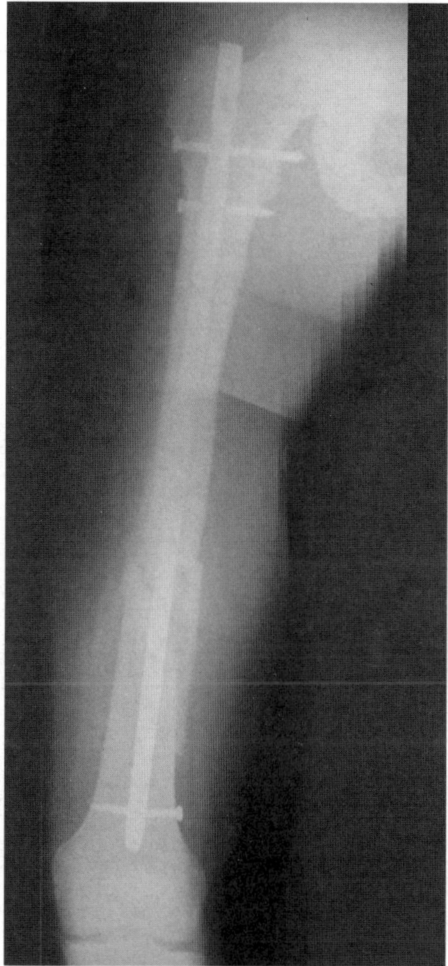

Figure 4.13: Femoral shaft fractures in adults are commonly treated with a locked intramedullary nail

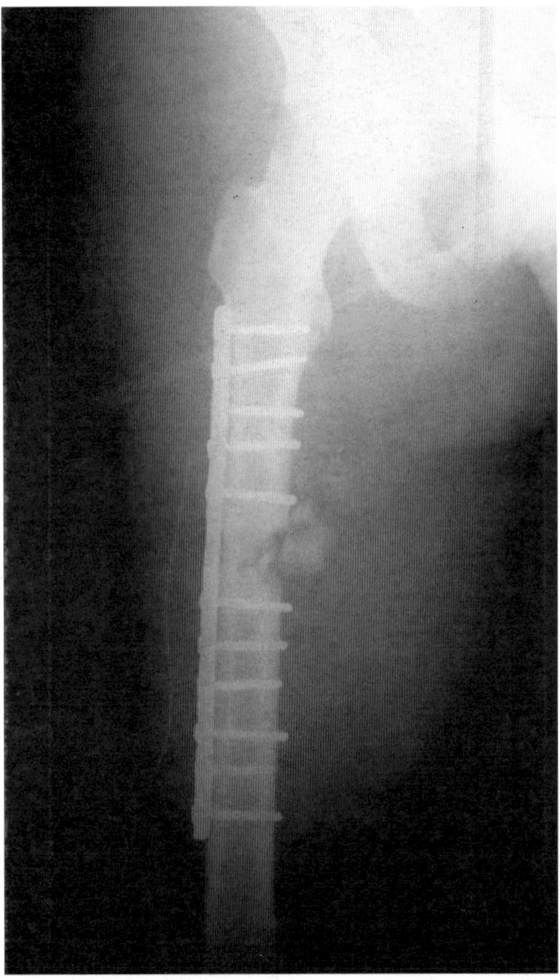

Figure 4.14: Femoral shaft fractures may be treated with open reduction and internal fixation in certain special situations (e.g. polytrauma, lack of facilities for interlocking nailing, etc.)

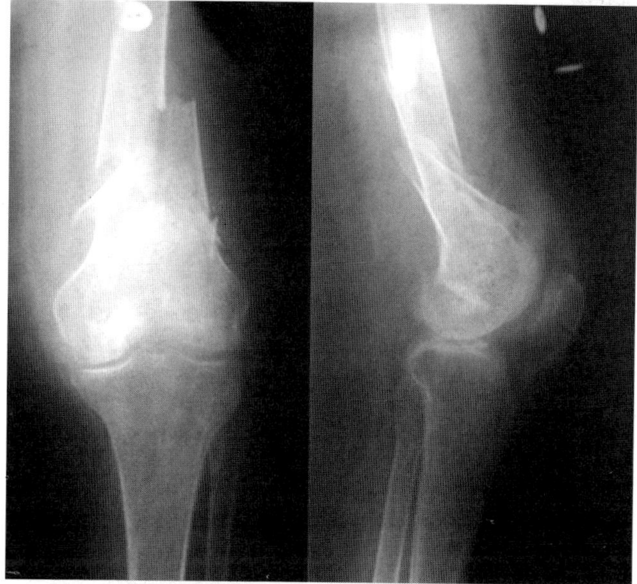

Figure 4.15: Supracondylar femoral fractures often require internal fixation. The distal fragment is flexed due to the unopposed pull of the gastrocnemius

are frequently associated with head, chest and pelvic injuries. Significant blood loss may be present. Intramedullary nailing is the commonest method of internal fixation for these fractures. Open reduction and internal fixation (plating) is indicated only in some cases (e.g. polytrauma). Conservative treatment (hip spica, traction, etc.) is preferred in children, especially if the alignment of the fracture is satisfactory.

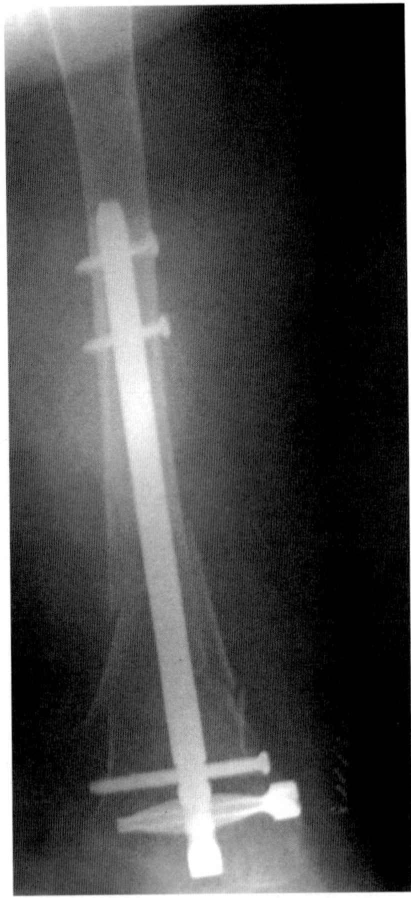

Figure 4.16: A supracondylar fracture of the femur stabilised with an interlocking retrograde nail

CHAPTER 5

Knee and Leg

TIBIAL PLATEAU FRACTURES

Fractures of the tibial plateau usually occur following high velocity injuries (e.g. road traffic accidents). Pain, swelling and haemarthrosis are common. Associated injuries to the collateral ligaments are common. Compartment syndrome is an important early complication. Undisplaced fractures are treated with a plaster cast or knee brace. Fractures associated with a significant depression of the articular surface are almost always treated with open reduction and internal fixation (Buttress plating and lag screws). Cancellous bone grafting from the iliac crest may also be necessary.

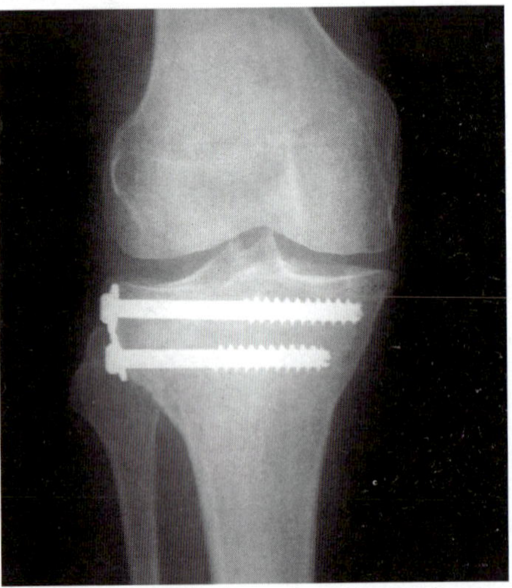

Figure 5.1: AP view of the knee showing a lateral tibial plateau fracture fixed with two cancellous lag screws

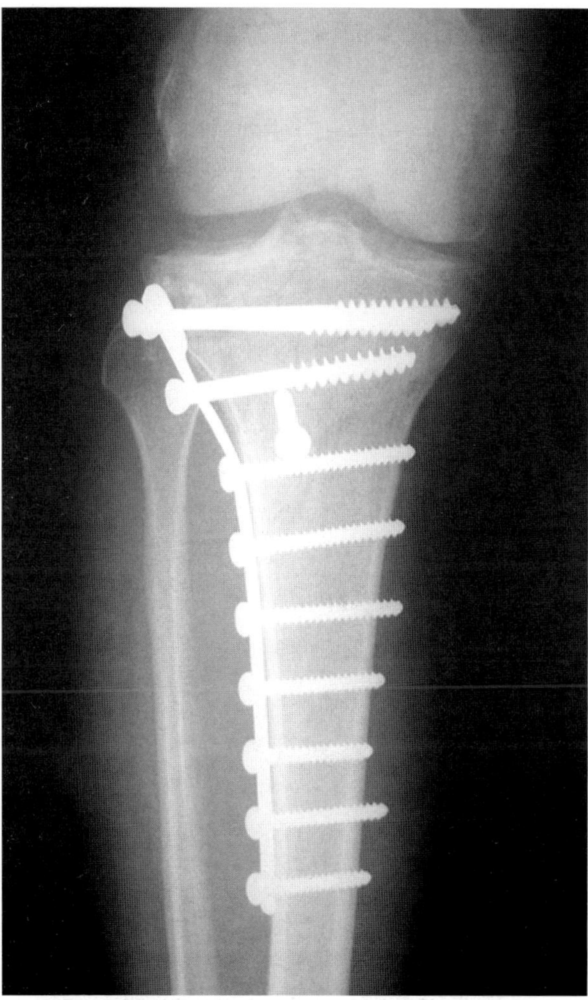

Figure 5.2: AP view of the knee showing a comminuted tibial plateau fracture treated with open reduction and internal fixation (Buttress Plating)

FRACTURES OF PATELLA

Patellar fractures commonly occur following direct trauma or as a result of a violent pull of the quadriceps muscle. The ability to actively extend and raise the leg should be assessed. Most undisplaced fractures in which the patient can demonstrate full active extension, may be treated conservatively (cylinder cast).

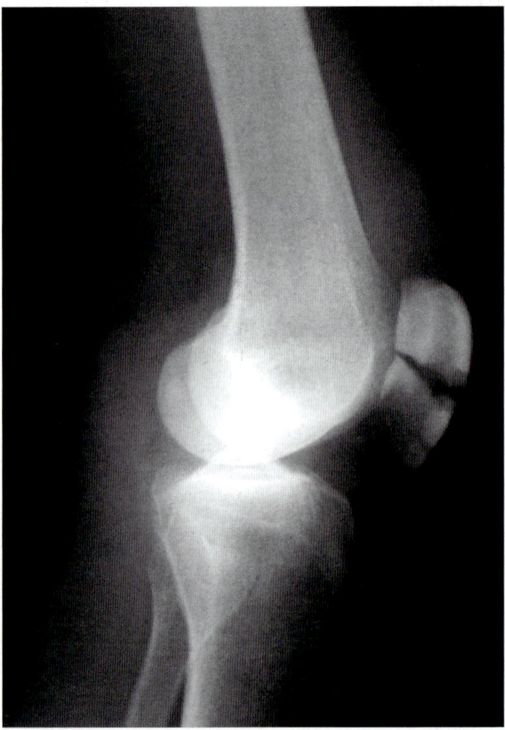

Figure 5.3: Lateral view of the knee showing a displaced fracture of the patella

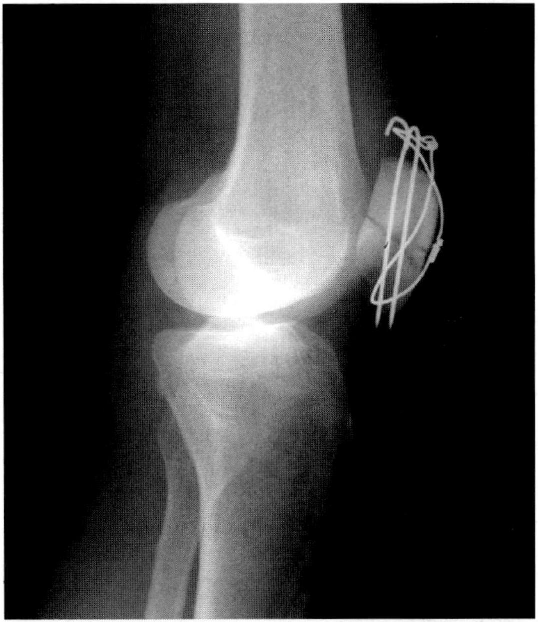

Figure 5.4: Lateral view of the knee showing a displaced patellar fracture treated with 'tension band (figure of eight) wiring'

However, if extensor mechanism is disrupted as in displaced fractures, operative treatment (e.g. Tension Band Wiring) is indicated. Knee stiffness is a common complication.

TIBIAL SHAFT FRACTURES

Most tibial shaft fractures occur following road traffic accidents or falls. Undisplaced fractures can be

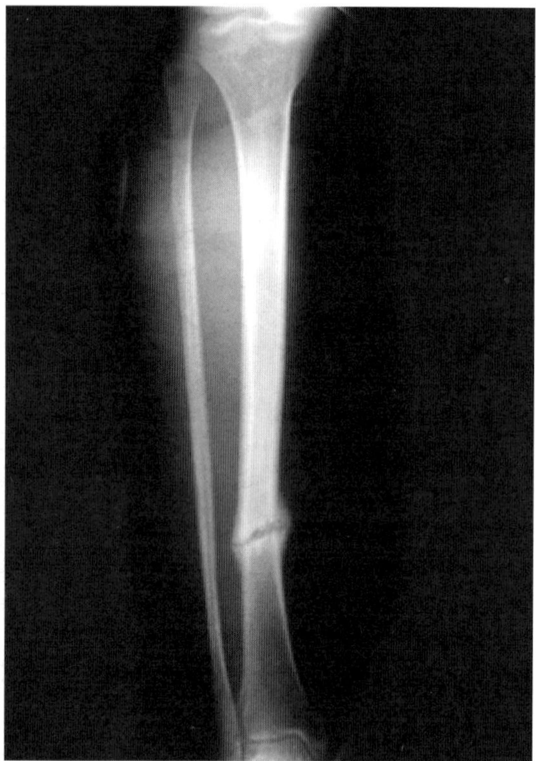

Figure 5.5: AP view of the leg showing a fracture of the shaft of the tibia showing callous formation following treatment with a plaster cast

satisfactorily treated with a 'long leg' cast. Intramedullary nailing is recommended for most displaced fractures which are otherwise difficult to control. Compartment Syndrome, malunion and non-union are important complications.

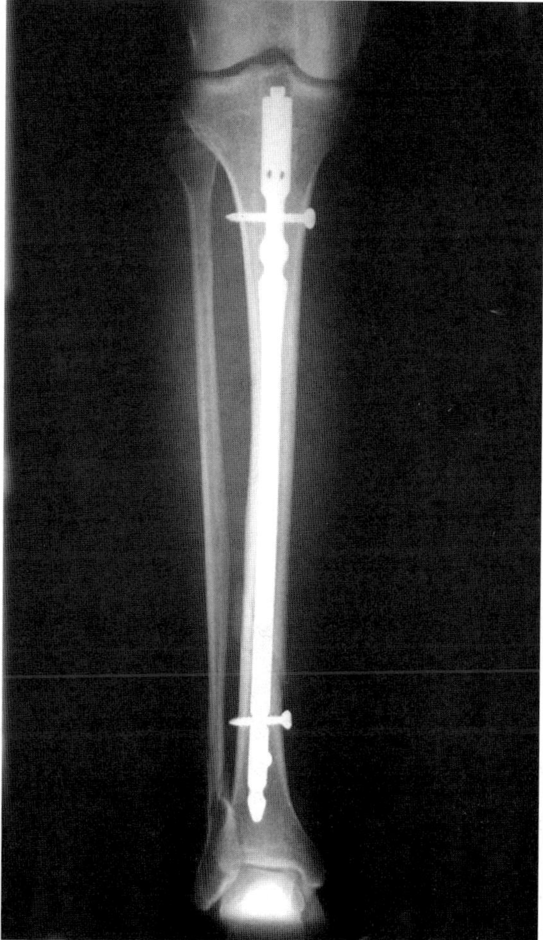

Figure 5.6: AP view of the leg showing a fracture of the tibial shaft treated with an intramedullary nail

CHAPTER 6

Ankle and Foot

ANKLE FRACTURES

Ankle fractures result from a combination of forces (eversion/inversion, pronation/supination and external rotation. The pattern of fracture depends upon the deforming force and position of the ankle at the time of injury. Severe disruptions to the ligaments are common. Most undisplaced fractures are treated satisfactorily with a plaster cast. Displaced fractures, especially those associated with disruption of the ankle mortise frequently require internal fixation (plating).

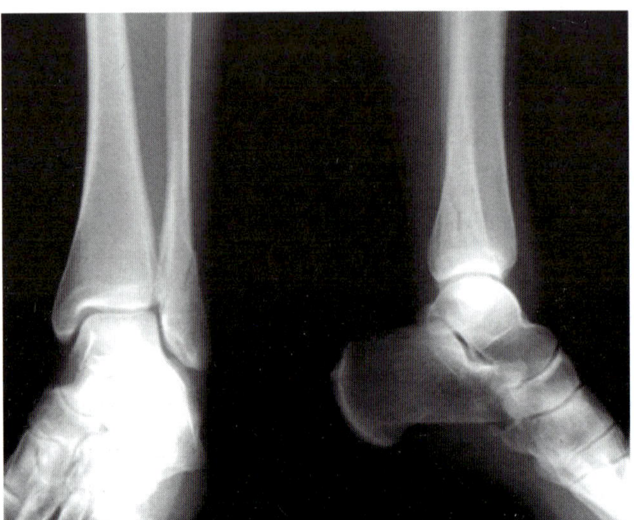

Figure 6.1: AP and lateral views of the ankle. Undisplaced or minimally displaced fractures of the lateral malleolus can be treated successfully without surgery if the ankle mortise is not disrupted

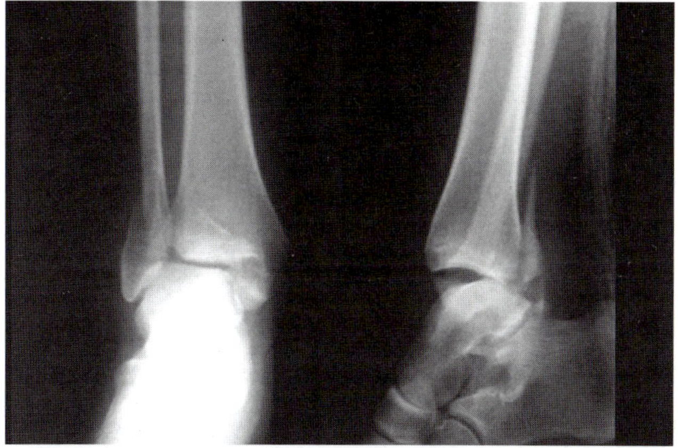

Figure 6.2: AP and lateral views of the ankle showing a displaced trimalleolar fracture

CALCANEAL FRACTURES

Fractures of the calcaneum usually occur following falls from heights. Associated injuries to the spine, opposite calcaneum, pelvis and ankle are common. The fracture may be intra- or extra-articular. Most undisplaced fractures are treated with cold compression, elevation and compression bandaging. Displaced fractures, especially those involving the articular surface are treated with internal fixation with reconstruction plates. Peroneal tendon impingement, osteoarthritis and bony spurs are important complications.

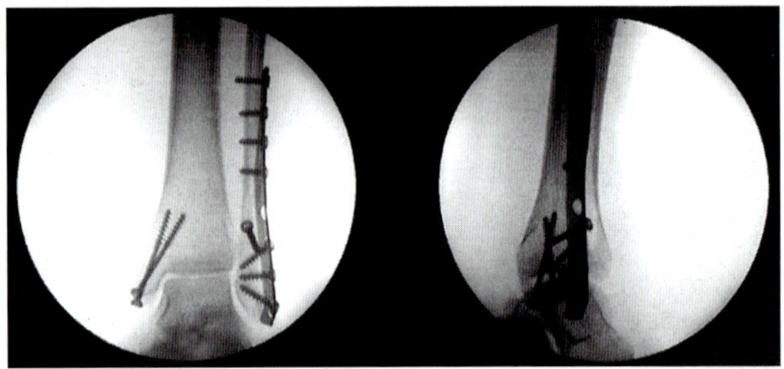

Figure 6.3: AP and lateral views of the ankle showing a displaced bimalleolar fracture fixed with plates and screws

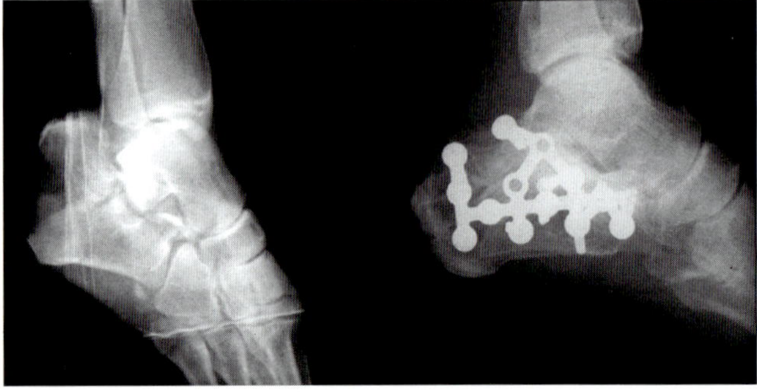

Figure 6.4: Lateral view of the ankle showing a severely comminuted fracture of the calcaneum stabilised with reconstruction plates

FRACTURES OF THE TALUS

Axial force in a dorsiflexed ankle, inversion/eversion or simple shear may be responsible for causing talar fractures. More than 50% fractures involve the neck of the talus. Talar neck fractures are commonly treated

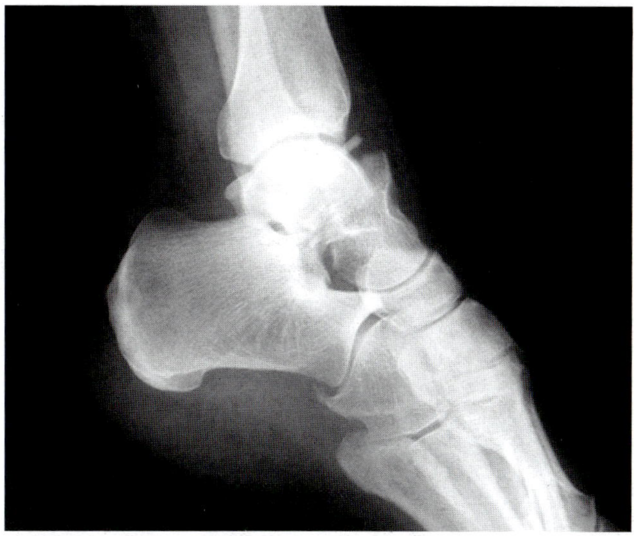

Figure 6.5: Lateral view of the ankle showing a displaced fracture of the neck of talus

with open reduction and internal fixation (screws). Undisplaced fractures of the lateral or posterior processes and of the body may be treated conservatively with a plaster cast.

METATARSAL FRACTURES

The most commonly involved metatarsal is the fifth.

A twisting force in the foot causes avulsion of the base (peroneus brevis attachment) of the fifth metatarsal (Jones' fracture). Most of these fractures are satisfactorily treated with a tubigrip or plaster cast.

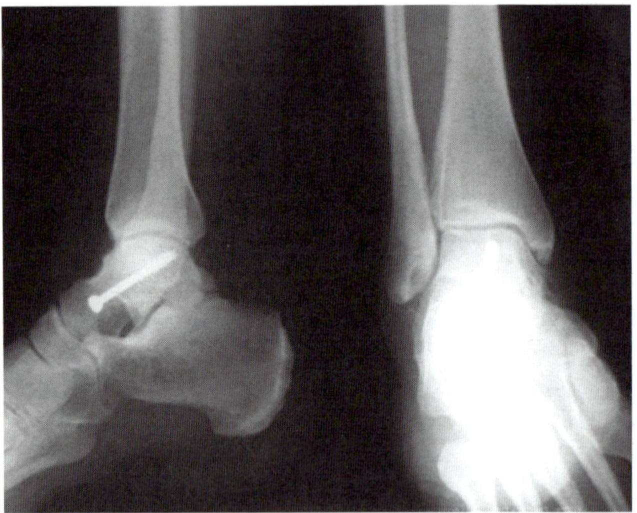

Figure 6.6: AP and lateral views of the ankle showing fixation of a talar neck fracture with a single screw

Two or more metatarsals may fracture following direct trauma (road traffic accidents, fall of heavy objects) often requiring manipulation and K-wiring for stabilisation. Disruptions of the tarsometatarsal joints (Lisfranc's injury), if present, require aggressive treatment with closed or open reduction and fixation (K-wire/screw).

TOE (PHALANGEAL) FRACTURES

Fractures of the phalanx are relatively minor injuries and can be satisfactorily treated conservatively with

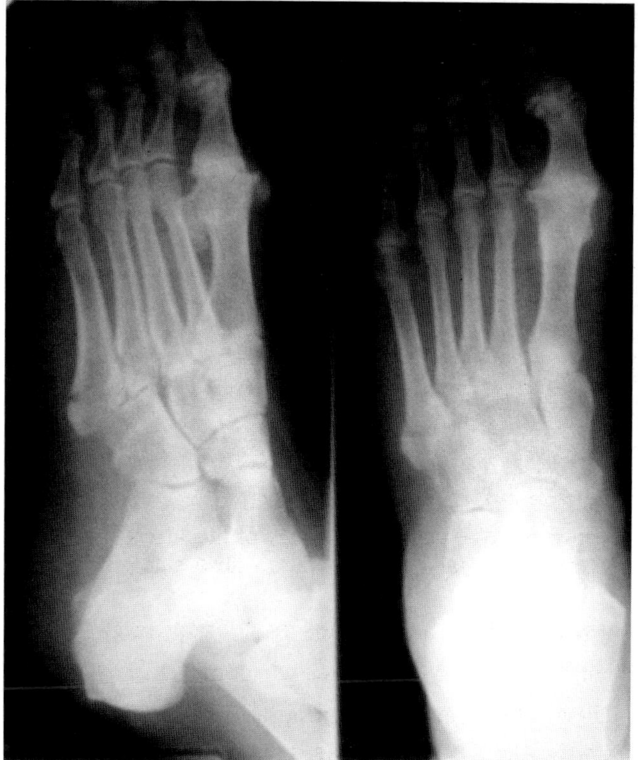

Figure 6.7: AP and oblique views of the foot showing an avulsion fracture of the base of the fifth metatarsal

'neighbour strapping'. However, occasionally, manipulation and fixation with K-wires or screws may be necessary, especially if there is severe rotational or angular deformity or intraarticular involvement.

Section 3
Spine

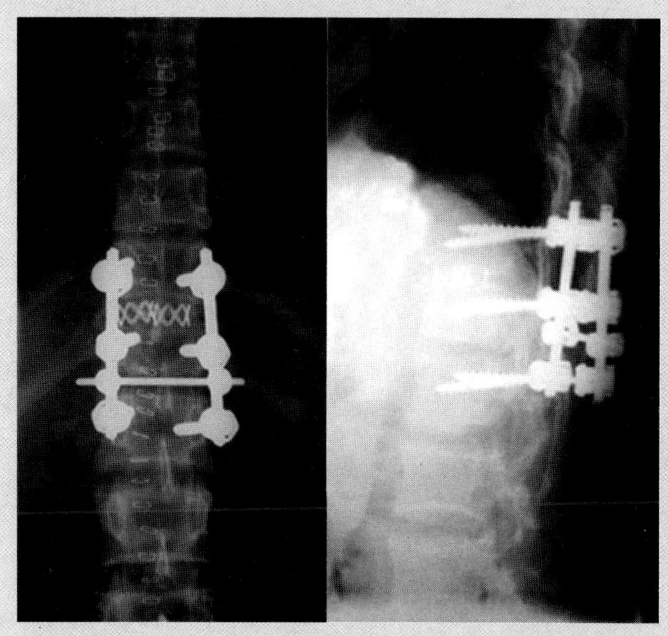

CHAPTER 7

Spine

INTRODUCTION

Injuries to the vertebral column usually result from violent falls and road traffic accidents. Wedge compression fractures of the dorsolumbar spine in the elderly age group following trivial falls are usually related to osteoporosis. However, in some cases they may represent a malignant metastatic process.

Injuries involving the neck require immediate cervical immobilisation. Serious airway compromise may be present. The patient should be managed according to the Advanced Trauma Life Support Guidelines [Management of **A**irway with cervical spine immobilisation, **B**reathing and **C**irculation (ABC)]. Other associated injuries (head, chest, pelvis etc) may also be present.

Spinal column injuries should be treated with caution. A complete neurological assessment is mandatory. The principles of 'in line immobilisation' and 'log roll' should be closely followed.

In general, all stable fractures are treated conservatively with early mobilisation. Braces and plaster jackets may be necessary in some cases. Unstable or potentially unstable fractures and those associated with neurological compromise are stabilised with internal fixation (e.g. pedicle screw fixation for dorsolumbar injuries).

IMPORTANT DEFINITIONS

Jefferson's Fracture

Burst fracture of the atlas (C1) ring resulting from a vertical compression injury.

Hangman's Fracture

Bilateral Pedicle fractures of the axis (C2) resulting from sudden hyperextension and distraction of the neck.

Clayshoveller's Fracture

Avulsion fracture of spinous processes of the lower cervical (usually C7) or upper thoracic vertebrae as a result of sudden hyperflexion of the neck.

Chance's Fracture (Seat belt type fracture)

Flexion-distraction injury involving the lumbar vertebrae with compression of the anterior and distraction of the posterior column.

Tear Drop Fracture

Avulsion fracture of the anteroinferior column of the cervical spine (usually C7).

Cauda Equina Syndrome

Compression of the lower lumbosacral roots by a fracture, prolapsed disc, abscess or tumour leading to saddle anaesthesia, numbness or weakness, bilateral radicular pain, loss of reflexes and impaired bowel and bladder function. Urgent spinal canal decompression plus/minus stabilisation is indicated.

Whiplash Injury

Hyperextension combined with flexion and rotation of the neck following rear low velocity motor vehicle collisions, sometimes, produces significant neck pain that may be associated with paraesthesia, dizziness, stiffness, etc. Loss of cervical lordosis may be the only positive finding on X-ray. Conservative treatment with painkillers and physical therapy is advised.

Although a whiplash injury is considered to be the commonest cause of chronic neck pain and stiffness following a vehicular collision, its role as a clinical entity is still controversial due to a high rate of successful litigations.

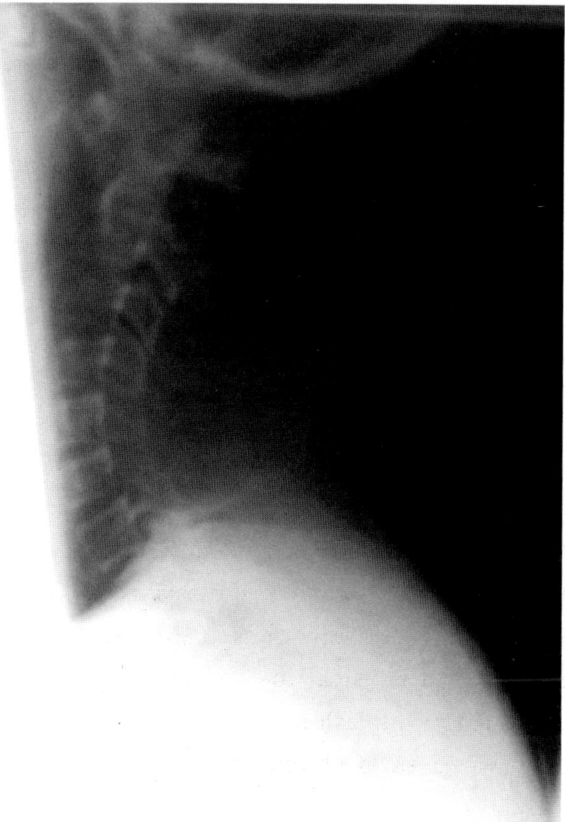

Figure 7.1: Lateral view of the cervical spine should include all the cervical vertebrae including the C7-T1 junction. Vertebral alignment, discontinuity and disc spaces should be carefully assessed

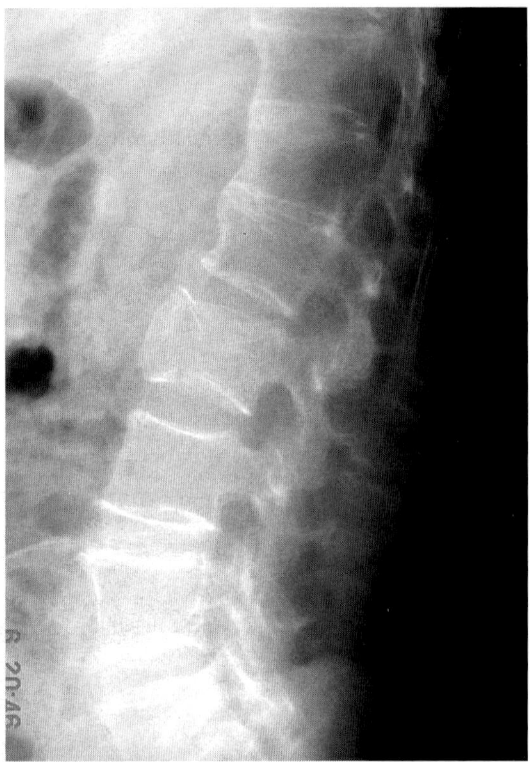

Figure 7.2: Lateral view of the lumbar spine showing a wedge compression fracture of L2

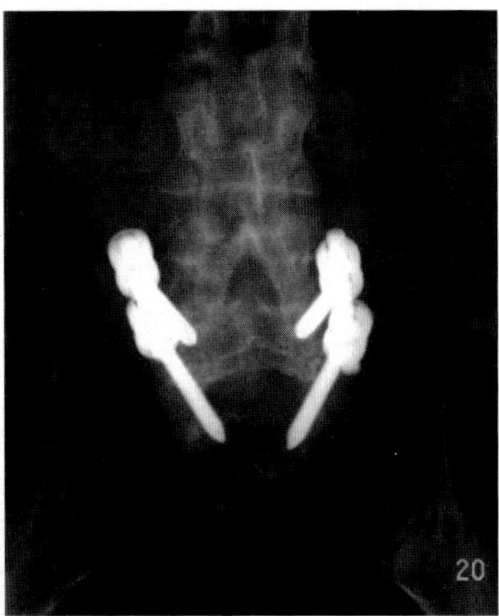

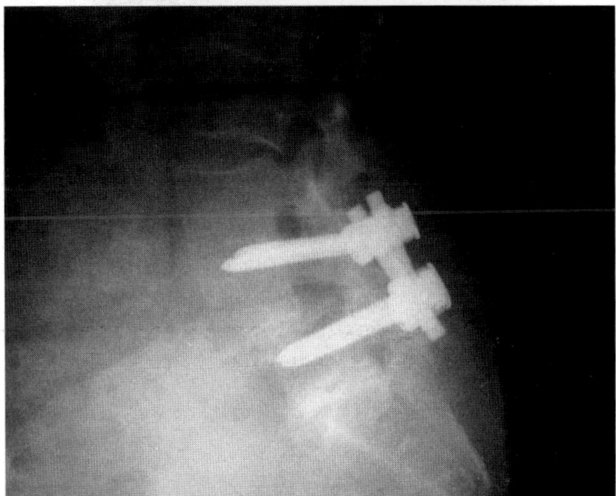

Figure 7.3: AP and lateral views of the dorsolumbar spine showing stabilisation with pedicle screws

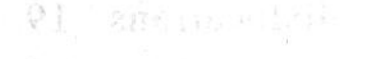

Index

A

Acromioclavicular joint injuries
- associated injuries 4
- internal fixation 6
- open reduction 6

Ankle fractures
- causes 68
- displaced trimalleolar fracture 69
- internal fixation 68
- treated with a plaster cast 68

Austin Moore's prosthesis 44

B

Barton's fracture 32, 35
Bipolar prosthesis 44
Boxer's fracture 36
Buttress plating 32, 35, 60

C

Calcaneal fractures
- associated injuries 69
- complications 69
- elevation and compression bandaging 69
- internal fixation with reconstruction plates 69, 70
- treated with cold compression 69

Clavicular fractures 4
- bone grafting 6
- clinical features 4
- internal fixation 4, 6
- open reduction 4, 6
- sling treatment 5

D

Diaphyseal fractures of the forearm bones 27
- flexible intramedullary nails 28
- open reduction and internal fixation 28, 29
- treated with an above elbow cast 28

Dinner fork deformity 32
Distal radius fractures 32, 34, 35
- Barton's fracture 33
- Chauffeur's fracture 33
- Colles fracture 32
- fixation with K-wires 35
- osteoporosis 32
- Smith's fracture 32
- treated with open reduction and internal fixation 32

E

Elbow dislocations 19

F

Figure of eight wiring 63
Fracture of the lateral condyle stabilised with K-wires 19

Fractures of patella
causes 62
complication 63
treated with cylinder cast 62
treated with tension band wiring 63
Fractures of the femoral shaft 52
associated injuries 57
causes 52
intramedullary nailing 57
open reduction and internal fixation 57
stabilised with an interlocking retrograde nail 58
stabilised with flexible intra-medullary nails 54
treated with a locked intra-medullary nail 55
treated with open reduction and internal fixation 56
treatment with hip spica, traction 57
unite with a plaster spica or traction 53
Fractures of the hip
femoral neck fractures 44
fixed with cannulated screws 44, 47
fixed with two cannulated screws 47
hemiarthroplasty 44, 46
hip screw fixation 44
important complications 44
intertrochanteric fracture 48
osteoporosis 44
Fractures of the lateral condyle 16
Fractures of the metacarpal 34, 37
internal fixation with K-wires 36
stabilised with two transverse K-wires 37
treated with neighbour strapping of the fingers 36
Fractures of the phalanx 72
fixation with K-wires 73
fixation with screws 73
treated with neighbour strapping of the fingers 72-73
Fractures of the talus
causes 70
treated with a plaster cast 71
treated with open reduction and internal fixation 71

H

Hip dislocations
causes 48
complications 52
fixation with a reconstruction nail 51
treatment with a dynamic hip screw 49
Humeral shaft fractures 10
complication 11
treated with bone grafting 13
treated with functional brace 10
treated with internal fixation 11
treated with intramedullary nailing 13
treated with plaster slab 10

I

Injuries to the vertebral column
Advanced Trauma Life Support Guidelines 78

associated injuries 78
braces and plaster jackets 78
cauda equina syndrome 80
causes 78
Chance's fracture 79
Clayshoveller's fracture 79
fracture of L2 82
Hangman's fracture 79
Jefferson's fracture 79
osteoporosis 78
pedicle screw fixation 78
stabilisation with pedicle screws 83
tear drop fracture 79
whiplash injury 80
Intercondylar fractures 16, 20
treated with internal fixation 20

J

Jones' fracture 71

L

Lag screws 60
Lisfranc's injury 72

M

Metatarsal fractures 71
causes 72
treated with a tubigrip or plaster cast 71
treated with open reduction and fixation 72

N

Nancy nails 28, 54
Neer's prosthesis 11

O

Olecranon fractures 21, 23, 24
fixation with a reconstruction plate 24
plating 21
treatment with tension band wiring 21, 23

P

Pelvic fractures 42
aggressive resuscitation 43
associated injuries 42
fixation with an external fixator 43
hypovolaemia 42
internal fixation 43
open book pelvic injury 42
osteoporosis 42
Phalangeal fractures 37
treated with neighbour strapping of the fingers 37
treated with two cross K-wires 38
Polytrauma 57
Principles of in line immobilisation 78
Principles of log roll 78
Proximal humeral fractures
associated injuries 9
ORIF/hemiarthroplasty 10
treated with collar and cuff sling 10

R

Radial head fractures 22, 26
associated injuries 22
Essex-Lopresti lesion 27

excision/prosthetic replacement 25
fixation with multiple screws 26
Galeazzi's fracture 27
greenstick fracture 27
Monteggia's fracture 25
nightstick fracture 27
open reduction and internal fixation 25

S

Scaphoid fractures 33
treated with percutaneous screws 33, 36
Seat belt type fracture 79
Shoulder dislocations 6
anterior dislocation of the humeral head 8, 9
associated injuries 8
disrupted acromioclavicular joint 7
hook plate 7
internal fixation 7
open reduction 7
Smith's fracture 32, 35
Supracondylar fractures 16, 18
complications 16
stabilised with K-wires 18

T

Thompson's prosthesis 44
Tibial plateau fractures
associated injuries 60
complication 60
fixed with two cancellous lag screws 60
treated with a plaster cast or knee brace 60
treated with open reduction and internal fixation 60, 61
Tibial shaft fractures
causes 63
complications 64
intramedullary nailing 64, 65
treated with a long leg cast 64
Transolecranon approach 17, 20
Triceps splitting approach 17

W

Whiplash injury 80